D1824687

BRAIN FIT!

How Smarter Thinking Can Save Your Brain

Dr. Jenny Brockis

To Jan
Best wishes,
Jenny
x

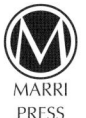

MARRI
PRESS

Brain Fit!

How Smarter Thinking Can Save Your Brain

Dr. Jenny Brockis, MB ChB FRACGP

First published November 2011

This edition published August 2013

Printed by Quality Press

Design and illustrations by Renée Fulton, rubi design

Edited by Jo-Anne Craine, Type A Creative, www.typeacreative.ca

ISBN 978-0-9871475-2-3

A CIP catalogue of this book is available from the National Library of Australia

DEDICATION

For Amanda

ACKNOWLEDGEMENTS

As with any project, taking the first flash of an idea to full fruition takes time, some effort and team work. Transforming my thoughts from my blog into a user- and reader-friendly guide to help show people that we all have the ability "to sculpt our own mind" has been a fun, sometimes challenging path.

My thanks start first with the wonderful tribe that makes up the Perth WA chapter of NSAA, fellow speakers and authors with messages of their own to share with the world. You all provided me with inspiration, support and encouragement. Special thanks go to Paula Smith, Julie Meek, David Beard, Jason Fox and David Price. You guys rock!

To Dr. Desi Silva, Liz Wright, Julie Taylor and Hayley Solich: I am so blessed to have your friendship. And where would I be without the best swimming coach in the world, Amanda? My number one fan, who has not only taught me how to swim but has been a driving force to encourage me to succeed in all of my endeavours.

Thanks go too, to my editor, Jo-Anne Craine at Type A Creative. You are a wonderful woman and I truly appreciate all the hard work you put into this manuscript.

And finally, I want to acknowledge my family. Without you by my side, none of this would have got off the ground. John, you provide unconditional love and support, picking me up when I fall down and helping to dust off my knees, so I can get up and get going again. And to Tom and Sophie, I love you so much.

FOREWORD

Whenever I tell someone about how little we know about dementia and the diseases that cause it, I'm met with disbelief.

It is difficult to comprehend how in an age of iPads and smartphones, we are no closer to knowing the exact cause of dementia. We can clone an animal, but we are decades away from finding a cure for dementia.

What we do know about some dementias are the risk factors; the variables which we can change to reduce our risk. Factors such as physical health, exercise and diet. This includes your mental fitness, which is distinct from mental health. Until we find a cure for dementia, prevention remains a priority, and increasing your brain fitness significantly reduces the risk of dementia.

There is truth to the saying that the brain is like a muscle and it needs to be exercised. Brain fitness is not just a diet, or an exercise, or a mental drill, or an attitude, but a combination of all of the above. A holistic approach to brain health is much more effective than focusing on any one factor by itself.

Dr Jenny Brockis is an expert in this field and a regular contributor to Alzheimer's Australia WA's quarterly magazine. Her advice on maintaining mental fitness is echoed in many of our information sheets.

The beauty of this book lies in its simplicity. The suggested actions are simple, straightforward and easy to implement, and are presented in a clear manner for readers to follow.

This book is a welcome guide to improving brain fitness and invaluable for anyone concerned for their health. I hope you find it as useful as I did.

Frank J Schaper

Chief Executive Officer

Alzheimer's Australia WA Ltd

CONTENTS

CHAPTER 1

BECOMING BRAIN FIT FOR LIFE

"Every man can, if he desires, become the sculptor of his own brain."

—Santiago Ramon y Cajal

We go to the gym, we watch our weight and eat sensibly, yet the one thing many of us often forget to do is to stretch our mental muscles and keep brain fit.

But if we are using our brains all the time in our busy lives, at work and at home, isn't all this mental activity enough?

The short answer is no. In the same way that being physically active does not always imply physical fitness, it's very similar for our brains.

How much time do we actually allocate to maintaining our brain fitness?

In reality, probably not much, yet it doesn't require a lot of time to make a significant difference to our brain health and fitness. The trouble is that we are often too busy to notice when we are working sub-optimally. It is only when the cracks really start to show that we stop and wonder why.

Like the time you forget an important client's name, or an appointment.

Or when you are unable to locate that urgent file your boss wanted 10 minutes ago; or when the deadline for submitting a tender is looming and you haven't allocated sufficient time to get the necessary legwork completed.

Don't you just love that sinking feeling when, just before going into a two-hour meeting, you open your inbox and 400 emails come flooding in, all needing your attention today? There is no end to the work pressures we face that break concentration and increase stress. What do you do when your child has a raging temperature and there is no one to take care of him at home? Does having your child at your workplace distract you from your ability to focus and pay attention?

These are common daily issues. Yet they can all have a significant impact on how we cope and survive our working day. Imagine if, by being more brain fit, these incidents were more easily manageable and did not impact your ability to perform as well as you wanted in your daily tasks.

Being brain fit means you can have improved attention, better memory skills, a greater capacity to think well and an increased ability to manage your stress levels. All of which is likely to produce an improvement in your work performance and overall happiness in life. When you are alert, happy and engaged, your productivity and creativity can soar.

When we are at work we rely on our brains to make good decisions, to have good recall, to be able to manage working relationships with staff and clients, to be focused, attentive and able to facilitate change.

Yet how often on a daily basis are our good intentions sabotaged by the brain drainers of fatigue, boredom, distractions, miscommunication and negative emotions?

Businesses are starting to recognise the importance of brain fitness to assist in the retention of staff, decreasing and reducing the amount of sick- and stress leave taken and thus boosting overall employee productivity and efficiency.

Being brain fit is good for everyone outside the workplace as well.

It means your mind is working optimally in all areas: having the emotional, cognitive and physical intelligence to think, feel and remember well.

Becoming brain fit is easy. We'll explore how a variety of influences and choices can affect your mental prowess. You will see how simple decisions you make in many aspects of your life play a part in elevating your overall brain fitness. Once you have become brain fit, you need to consciously take steps to maintain or further improve those areas you think could do with a bit of extra help. As we can only maintain physical fitness by continuing to exercise, it also holds true for our brains.

There is no quick fix, pill or supplement that is instantly going to turn you into a super intelligent MENSA member, although you may notice your brain is working a lot better for you when you start enjoying clear thinking and an improved ability to pay attention as a result of becoming brain fit.

In choosing to implement your own personal program of brain fitness, the dividends will pay off now as your level of brain fitness improves and will also pay off for the future. Studies have shown that by engaging in mentally stimulating activities, we build up our cognitive reserve, which protects our brain from the effects of age-related cognitive decline and dementia.

One of the greatest things you can do for your mental well-being is to be able to use your brain effectively throughout your life and enjoy a brain-healthy lifestyle.

The human brain can face a number of hurdles over one's lifespan, including brain injury and neurodegenerative disease.

The biggest factor in developing Alzheimer's disease and dementia is, simply, ageing. It's something none of us can avoid. We can't change our genetic predisposition, either.

However, we can control our environment and that has a significant impact on our overall health and well-being. It can make a difference to our gene expression – which genes are expressed, and when.

Having a family history of Alzheimer's disease or dementia may put you in a higher risk category but it is not a forgone conclusion that you will also be affected. There is so much that can make a difference to help us preserve our intellect and the best time to be looking after our brains is actually all throughout our lives.

And it is never too late to make a start.

With Brain Fit!, you can dip in and out of the different topics and tips to determine and develop your own brain fitness program, ensuring all areas of nutrition, stress management, mental activity and exercise are covered.

Happy dipping!

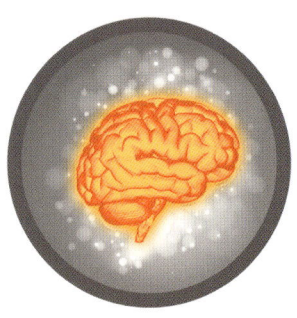

CHAPTER 2

KNOW YOUR BRAIN

WHAT ARE THE RISK FACTORS FOR DEMENTIA?

The original idea behind this book was to provide information and insight into how your lifestyle choices can make a significant difference to how well your brain works.

The risk of developing Alzheimer's disease or other dementia is ever-present, particularly as a primary factor is ageing. None of us can stop getting older. However, your actions now in adopting a healthy brain lifestyle and maintaining it throughout your life allows you to protect your brain as best you can from cognitive decline and impairment.

All of the lifestyle factors discussed in this book are under our control, to some degree. It is up to each one of us to be responsible for our own brain and to look after it as if it were the Crown Jewels. I sometimes describe this as keeping all our precious marbles highly polished.

THE ROLE OF AGE

At the turn of the 20th century, the average lifespan for Europeans was around 50 years. Today many of us will easily exceed three score years and ten (70). We see increasing numbers of people reaching 100. Unfortunately for some of us, our longevity will be accompanied by the onset of cognitive impairment and dementia.

Alzheimer's disease typically starts after the age of 65 except in the case of a very small number of people who carry what is known as an autosomal dominant gene mutation. These people will develop early onset dementia, i.e., before the age of 65.

The gene known as Apolipoprotein E4 is associated with a higher risk of susceptibility to Alzheimer's disease. However, the vast majority of people with Alzheimer's disease (around 60%) do not carry this gene. Testing is available but not currently recommended. Carrying the gene does not necessarily imply you will definitely express the gene and develop Alzheimer's.

It is, however, accepted that having a first-degree family member with Alzheimer's does increase your relative risk by two to three times the standard rate. Having two first-degree family members increases your relative risk by eight times. Another special group at higher risk of dementia include people with Down syndrome. Studies have suggested that between 50-70% of people with Down syndrome will develop dementia after the age of 60 years.

The indigenous population of Australia in addition to their many other health disadvantages, including having a shorter lifespan, have a rate of dementia that is 4.8 times higher than for non-indigenous Australians.

Currently the prevalence of dementia in Australia is 1.7% of men and 1.3% of women aged 65 to 69 years, rising to 37% of men and 47% of women aged 95 years or more. This is based on statistics from Access Economics 2009.

PREVALENCE OF DEMENTIA IN AUSTRALIA

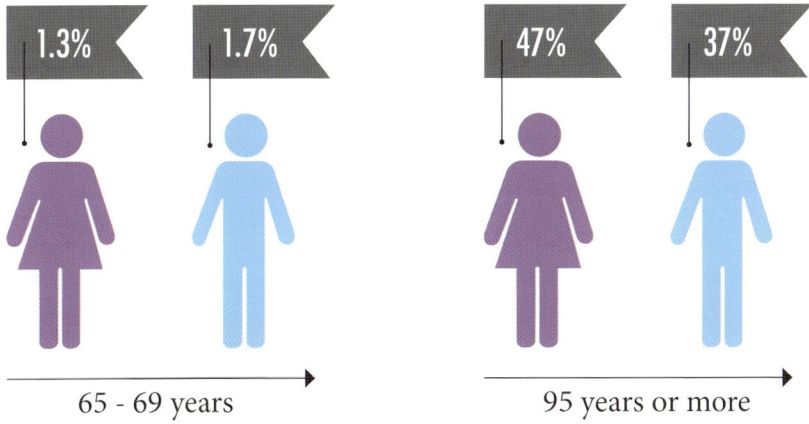

65 - 69 years   95 years or more

In 2010, the total number of people living in the world with dementia was estimated at 35.6 million, equivalent to 0.5% of the world's total population. This is expected to double over the next twenty years to 65.7 million by 2030, largely as a result of our ageing society. By 2050 the estimate rises to 115.4 million people worldwide.

By 2050 there will be nearly 2 billion people in the world aged over 50 years of age.

Dementia is **NOT** a normal part of ageing.

With the number of people being diagnosed with some form of dementia standing at roughly 7.7 million per year this is equivalent to one new person being diagnosed **every four seconds.**

ESTIMATED PEOPLE LIVING WITH DEMENTIA WORLDWIDE

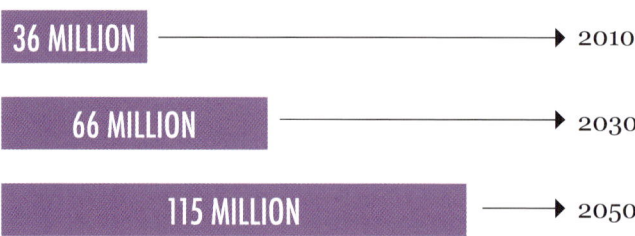

36 MILLION → 2010

66 MILLION → 2030

115 MILLION → 2050

The cost of caring for someone with dementia cannot be counted in terms of dollars alone, although the cost is huge. A person diagnosed with Alzheimer's disease or other form of dementia is likely to be cared for at home in the early to moderate stages of the disease and can be expected to live for an average of 10 years – a lengthy period of time for ongoing and continual support and care.

The World Dementia Report divides these costs into three separate entities that vary according to the wealth and support structures of different countries. In Australia, a wealthy country, the costs are roughly divided as follows:

- Informal care costs provided by family members = 45% of total costs
- Formal social care costs where providers assist with laundry shopping and other daily activities of living = 40% of total costs
- Direct medical costs = 15% of total costs

Currently, families provide much of the informal care. The concern is for those families where the parents are now middle-aged and working to support their children, and in addition supporting their ageing, and in some instances ailing parents, both financially, physically and emotionally. This generation is becoming known as the "sandwich generation" because they are working to support both the younger and the older generations.

THE ROLE OF LIFESTYLE FACTORS

We can't change our genes, but we can change the way we choose to eat, work, exercise and think.

The evidence from research is now consistently showing that we will have either a higher or lower risk of developing Alzheimer's disease or other form of dementia through the choices we make over the course of our lifespans.

The first step in cultivating and enjoying a healthier brain for as long as possible is to have the knowledge and understanding of these lifestyle factors.

Lifestyle factors we can influence:

HYPERTENSION
SMOKING PHYSICAL ACTIVITY OR EXERCISE
MENTAL ACTIVITY AND CHALLENGE
SOCIALISATION OBESITY
ATTITUDE
DIABETES STRESS AND DEPRESSION
HIGH CHOLESTEROL
ALCOHOL DIET

In this book I will distil and share some of the evidence from research and clinical trials that clearly convey how modifying one's lifestyle can produce positive change and allow you to have a healthier brain.

There is currently no cure for dementia. But if we can delay or defer the clinical onset of clinical symptoms of dementia by five years through lifestyle change, it is projected that the incidence of dementia expected in 2050 could be halved. How would you like to reduce your risk by 50%?

In 2012, there were approximately 280,000 people in Australia living with dementia. Because of our ageing population, this is expected to increase to over 1.13 million by 2050. The possibility of being able to achieve a 50% reduction in those projections of the number of people likely to develop Alzheimer's or dementia, along with reducing the burden to society, is something I believe we cannot ignore and need to focus our attention on, starting today.

SMARTER THINKING: We cannot stop the clock or change our genes. What we do have, though, is the ability through our lifestyle choices to influence those modifiable factors that determine our relative risk of cognitive decline or dementia.

YOUR AMAZING PLASTIC BRAIN

Along with all the amazing new technologies we have been enjoying over the last couple of decades, medical research and neuroscience now provides an incredible amount of knowledge and greater understanding of how the brain works. There is still an incredible amount that we don't understand as yet. However, we are in a fantastic position to know that each and every one of us has capacity, if we so choose, to improve and maintain our brain functions as best we can over the course of our lifetime.

In the early 1980s, medical students were still being taught that the brain was hard-wired; incapable of change. The concept of neuroplasticity was unheard of.

We now know that far from being hard-wired, the brain is dynamic. Our brain cells or neurons are constantly re-wiring, forming new neural pathways and pruning ones no longer required in response to the barrage of incoming sensory information one's brain receives every day.

We have between 85 and 100 billion brain cells. Each one is capable of forming 10,000 or more connections with other brain cells through synapses. Each brain cell has multiple small branches, or dendrites. At the end of the dendrites where it meets the dendrite of a neighbour, there is a small space called the synaptic cleft. When an excitatory or inhibitory electrical impulse travels down a dendrite, neurochemicals stored at the terminal are released into this space, to be taken up by receptors of the neighbouring dendrite terminal. This allows the message to then be passed along.

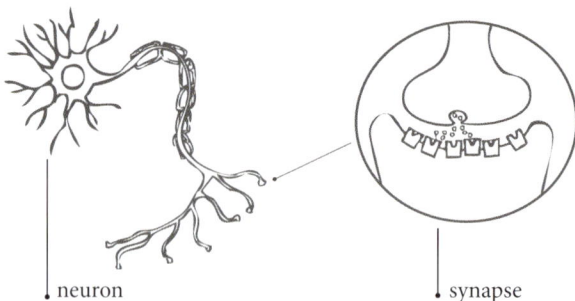

neuron   synapse

Your brain is a multiplicity of electrical signals and a warm bath of neurochemicals allowing you to form thoughts, keep memories, pay attention, know where you are in space, be able to reason, plan and speak ... to name just some of its capabilities.

Plastikos. It's the Greek word meaning mouldable or malleable. When we talk of having a plastic brain, we mean it is changeable. Neuroplasticity is the concept that the brain is constantly changing, remodelling our neural pathways in response to the sensory information it receives.

We also have neurogenesis: the production of new neurons or brain cells. A couple of highly specialised areas in the brain have this capability, one of which is the hippocampus, and another area that's associated with the olfactory bulbs, which we use for our sense of smell. Our brains can produce these new brain cells throughout our lives. If conditions are conducive, these will survive, mature and be incorporated into our existing brain circuitry. Certain brain chemicals enhance their survival and physical exercise has been shown to stimulate the production of these sustaining brain chemicals, and enhance neurogenesis.

OUR BRAINS CHANGE AS WE AGE

Our speed of processing starts to slow down. We don't actually start to notice this until we are in our 40s and 50s. It's that conscious awareness that we are not quite as sharp as we used to be; we forget things more easily or misplace items we absentmindedly put down.

Our brains are shrinking. Not by much, around 0.2% per year, but there is a very gradual loss of brain volume. Having the capacity to build new connections between our remaining brain cells is important as we age, to enable us to keep our cognition intact and allow us to continue to take in new information and lay down new memories.

What our brains gain as we age, though, is the wisdom of experience. We are better able to cope with some of life's challenges because we can draw upon our previous experiences and memory. We stress less about certain issues and are often happier because of this as well. Age can bring greater contentment with our lot.

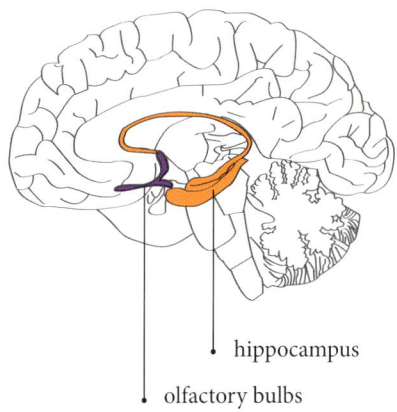

hippocampus

olfactory bulbs

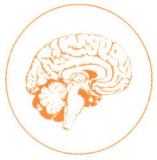

SMARTER THINKING: Having a plastic brain enables us to be lifelong learners. Ageing may slow down a few processes but we retain the ability to keep forming new connections, strengthening the neural pathways that allow us to keep our cognition intact. Continuing to engage in opportunities to learn new things helps us to maintain our brains.

COGNITIVE DECLINE: IS IT INEVITABLE?

The short answer is no.

One of the biggest issues I believe we face in society today is getting the message out that, yes, there is a tsunami of dementia approaching as a large segment of our population is ageing.

The good news is that the risk of developing dementia can be reduced by looking at our lifestyle and health behaviours.

But (and it's a big but), the vast majority of people remain unaware that they already have the power to reduce their own risk. Nearly half of the Australian population either don't know or don't know how.

In Australia, we already have around 280,000 people living with dementia and 1,300 new cases being diagnosed every week. For every one person living with the disease there are family members affected also, as they have to provide care and support for that person.

WE ALREADY HAVE OVER A QUARTER OF A MILLION PEOPLE IN AUSTRALIA LIVING WTH DEMENTIA

Take a look at the migration figures of people moving into different states each week. For example, there are currently about 1,000 people moving to the state of West Australia every week. That means more people nationally are being diagnosed with dementia each week than there are new migrants moving to W.A.

- It is anticipated that by 2050, there will be 7,400 people newly diagnosed with dementia each week.

- How are we going to cope with the significant economic and social burden?

- Worldwide, the global cost of dementia in 2010 was U.S. $604 billion. That is more than 1% of the global GDP.

- If dementia was a country, it would now have the world's 18th largest economy.

- Dementia costs exceed both Wal-Mart's annual revenue of U.S. $414 billion and Exxon Mobil's revenue of U.S. $311 billion.

- The number of people expected to have dementia is estimated to double by 2030 and possibly triple by 2050.

Cognitive decline is not an inevitable part of ageing.

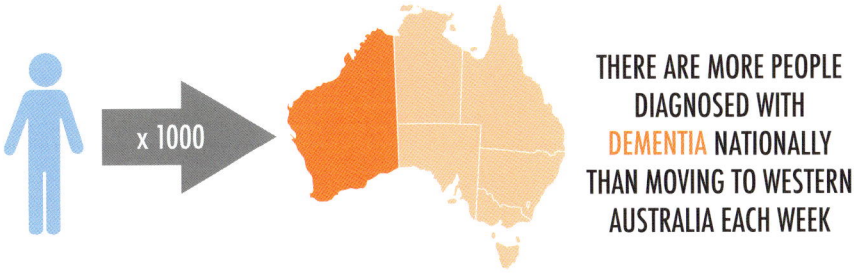

THERE ARE MORE PEOPLE DIAGNOSED WITH DEMENTIA NATIONALLY THAN MOVING TO WESTERN AUSTRALIA EACH WEEK

We can all aim to lower our risk of developing dementia in the following ways:

 Eating a healthy diet that includes lots of green leafy vegetables, red- skinned fruits, fish, nuts and dark chocolate

 Taking part in regular physical activity at least three times a week

 Stimulating our brains with new learning

 Not smoking

 Adopting a positive attitude towards healthy ageing

 Being involved in social activities

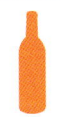 Drinking less alcohol

 Protecting our brains from injury

It's not rocket science.

We know what's good for us. We just have to do it. Perhaps that is the greatest challenge for us all.

The reality is that we are all likely to be touched by dementia in some shape or form, whether as a diagnosis for ourselves or through our involvement caring for a family member or friend.

The time to take action is now. The more we can protect ourselves by choosing to improve our lifestyle and make the healthy choices, the greater our chances of maintaining a healthy brain.

So what are you going to choose?

OUR ENVIRONMENT INFLUENCES OUR GENES

Recent studies prove that environmental factors can lead to changes in gene expression (without altering the genetic code), which can be passed on to successive generations.

Hang on a minute, you might argue, we have adhered to the Darwinian theory for 150 years. It proposed that evolution takes place slowly over many generations and is based on survival of the fittest. Changes in the evolutionary process are, therefore, slow.

The research indicates that the conditions your parents live under, can influence your health prior to your birth and also into your own adulthood.

So where does this new evidence come from that suggests the lifestyle choices we make today not only influence our risk factors for disease in ourselves, but also for our future children and grandchildren?

Welcome to the world of epigenetics.

Epigenetics is not new. Scientists have been exploring these concepts since the 1970s, piecing together information that supports the concept that the conditions that your parents live under can influence your health prior to your birth and also into your own adulthood.

Our genes contain our unique individual DNA.

On the top of our genes we have what is called an epigenome and it is this which influences our genes; by switching certain genes on or off, or being expressed strongly or weakly.

What is emerging is that diet and stress levels (and other lifestyle and environmental factors) can influence the epigenome and make a difference to the gene expression from one generation to another.

What does this all mean?

If we (that's you and me), choose to overeat, become obese or smoke, the epigenomes on our genes will cause the genes for obesity to be strongly expressed and the genes for lifespan to be more weakly expressed. This can be passed on to our kids and grandkids, making them at risk for disease and early death.

The potential for understanding how epigenetics can influence DNA and our future health is only just beginning.

In the future it may be possible to manipulate epigenetic markers and develop drugs that will be used to treat certain illnesses by either turning down the expression of genes we don't want expressed or enhancing expression of those we do.

The implication for treatments of disease such as certain cancers or Alzheimer's gives great hope.

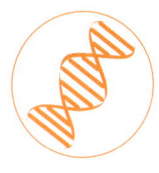

SMARTER THINKING: While we cannot change our genetic predisposition, we can influence our environment through lifestyle choices. These can exert an effect on our genes, influencing their actual, or timing of, expression. Our lifestyle choices today can impact the future health of our children and our children's children, through the influence our choices make on our epigenome.

CHAPTER 3

THE FOUR KEY ELEMENTS

So what are the fundamental elements to becoming brain fit? You might think that the workings of the brain are so complex you may never understand how best to keep it in top working order.

It's true, the brain is a miraculous and astounding thing, and scientists and doctors are learning more about it every day. The beauty of all this research means that by knowing how it functions, we better understand how to take care of it.

REMEMBER YOUR NAME®

As a doctor with expertise and an insatiable curiosity in this specialty, I am often asked to translate the medical jargon to my patients in a way they can apply the information to their daily lives.

There is so much information now available to us, providing greater understanding and insight into how our human brain works. But the sheer volume of information can be overwhelming. Every week new studies are published, some add new pieces of information, some support other findings and some will contradict. It can all get very confusing to be able to determine what exactly is relevant to us as individuals looking to understand our own brains better and improve brain function.

From my scientific and medical reading, and my writing of blog articles, I have attempted to filter down, clarify, define and organise the many factors, influences and information into four key components.

It's as easy as remembering your NAME®:

Nutrition; Attitude; Mental Challenge; and Exercise.

Nutrition
Feeding your brain with good nutrition allows it to work at its best.

Attitude
Learning good work/life integration and keeping stress under control keeps our brain cells happy.

Mental Challenge
Using our mental muscles allows us to keep learning.

Exercise
Doing some physical exercise actually helps keep your brain fit too.

By including all the elements from NAME®, you can develop your brain to achieve its peak performance and become brain fit!

The inter-relationship of these four elements enables you to strengthen your brain fitness muscles, which affect:

- Attention
- Memory
- Planning and organising skills
- Motor coordination
- Auditory, language and visual skills

REMEMBER YOUR NAME®

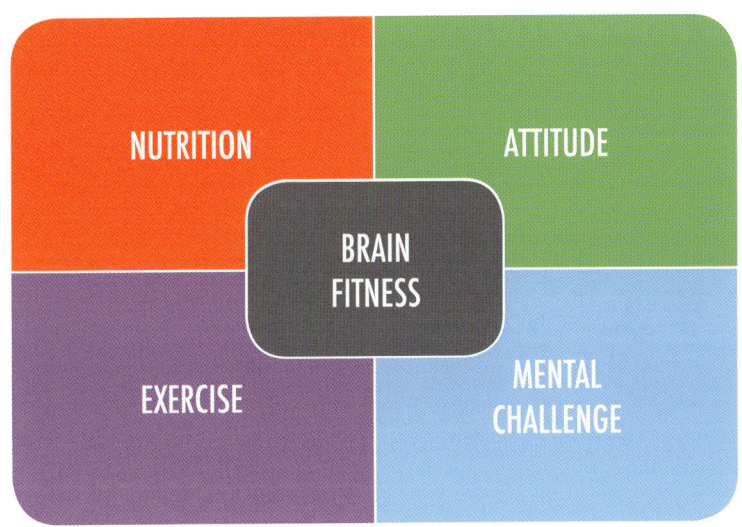

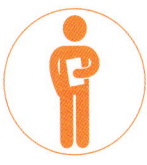 ***SMARTER THINKING:*** *As with any fitness program, it's necessary to cover all the basics so you can determine your current reality before moving on to identify which areas may need more attention. You can then design the most appropriate program for you, with help if needed; whether it is with a personal trainer, a coach or an accountability buddy.*

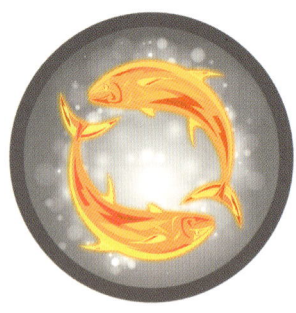

CHAPTER 4

NUTRITION: FEED YOUR BRAIN

It may only comprise a relatively small component of the body as a whole but in energy terms, the brain is an extremely hungry organ.

On average the human brain consumes 20% of the body's daily energy. It takes a lot of energy to think!

WHEN TO EAT

It is essential to provide the brain with sufficient, good quality nutrients to feed the demand and to help our brain cells reach and function at their optimum levels. Moreover, the brain likes a steady flow of nutrients, so eating little and often suits our brains better than having a couple of big meals intermittently.

REGULAR MEALS ARE ESSENTIAL

One of the biggest mistakes people make in terms of feeding their brains is skipping breakfast. The breakfast cereal adverts remind us that kids who don't eat breakfast get the "fuzzies" mid-morning. They seem unable to pay as much attention in class and they can't as effectively process the information they are being taught. Conversely, kids who do eat breakfast have been shown in studies to perform better in class tests, work better overall in the classroom and demonstrate fewer behavioural problems.

It is no different for us as adults. I know I get a little cranky when I get hungry and am less able to focus on the task at hand. Without fuel to kick-start your day you are not going to perform at your best. You have already been fasting overnight while asleep, so your body and mind are ready to receive some nourishment.

If you really can't face food first thing, then you can have a liquid breakfast in the form of a smoothie. But there is no substitute for a proper breakfast: wholegrain cereals or breads, a piece of fresh fruit and ideally, some protein. Eggs are a fabulous way to start your day as they are packed full of protein and choline (an ammonium salt in the vitamin B family, which your brain loves).

Not to sound like your mother, but she was right. Just eat something!

And what about lunch? In our busy lives, it is all too easy to work through the lunch break and deny one's brain the sustenance it needs. Without food our concentration drops off, we are more likely to make errors and our efficiency declines.

Additionally, as your blood sugar drops even lower, you may notice (or those around you will) yourself becoming more cranky and irritable. Those negative thinking patterns hinder brain performance even more.

So do yourself a favour. Stop! Enjoy your lunch. Your brain will thank you for it.

THE MID-AFTERNOON CRAVINGS: FRIEND OR FOE?

Another time of the day that can be an issue in terms of how well we are thinking and performing is mid-to-late afternoon. (Especially if we didn't stop for a proper lunch.) We've been busy all day and energy levels are starting to drop off but it's not time for dinner yet. This is the time we are most likely to reach for a quick sugary snack, biscuit or chocolate bar.

What we choose to eat now can have a dramatic effect on our brains.

If we choose a high sugar, high fat snack, our brains receive a sudden energy surge as the body's blood sugar levels are quickly boosted. This then triggers the pancreas gland in the abdomen to release the hormone insulin.

Insulin is responsible for regulating the body's blood sugar level and keeping it stable. The insulin quickly brings the blood sugar down to a more appropriate level but unfortunately in its enthusiasm it often overshoots. So two hours after that sugar snack, our blood sugar levels have plummeted into our boots. We end up more fatigued, cranky and hungrier than before, and our thinking skills decline.

Good brain food snacks include a handful of nuts, such as almonds or walnuts. People often worry that eating nuts will make them fat. In fact, eating a handful of protein-rich nuts allows your brain and appetite to be satisfied more quickly and for longer than eating carbohydrate. So unless you're eating half a kilo of nuts at a time, this is unlikely to cause issues with weight. Other alternatives include yoghurt, fruit, and a sandwich or wrap with some protein, which takes the body longer to break down. The brain still receives the nutrients and energy it needs but in a more sustainable way that will allow us to think well right up until the end of our working day.

Dinner is often the opportunity for families and couples to sit down together, talk over the day's events and wind down after a busy day. For many of us it is also likely to be the biggest meal of the day. Especially if breakfast and lunch were rushed and small.

"Eat breakfast like a king, lunch like a prince and dinner like a pauper."

There is a saying that we should "eat breakfast like a king, lunch like a prince and dinner like a pauper." However, in modern life many of us actually do the opposite. It makes more sense, though, to eat more during the day when we are at our most active. Eating a heavy meal or eating late in the evening means we are loading our bodies and brains at the wrong time. Excess nutrients not burnt off can contribute to weight gain. So ensure you eat a healthy dinner with plenty of vegetables, some lean protein and carbohydrates.

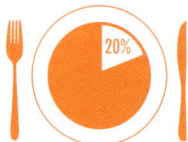

SMARTER THINKING: *: The brain is a greedy organ demanding 20% of the body's daily energy intake. It likes to receive a constant supply of nutrients in order to work at its best and our food choices also contribute to how well our brains will work for us.*

BEST BRAIN FOODS

Researchers and neuroscientists have discovered a lot more about the components of many different foods, including which ones are particularly good at helping our brain cells function at their best.

There are many supplements advertised as well. However the best combinations of antioxidants are still found in fresh (organic if available) fruit and vegetables. Nutritional manufacturers can combine different vitamins, minerals and herbs but none have been able to copy the synergistic effect of the various micronutrients that are found in our foods.

There is a time and a place for supplements as a result of deficiency, illness or poor diet but they should never be a substitute for the food we eat.

FOLLOWING A BRAIN HEALTHY DIET

"You are what you eat."

—Albert Signorella, DDS

In recent years there has been enormous interest in the results of nutritional research, looking to identify the potential cognitive benefits of consuming particular foods and whether we should be including more or less of them in our diets.

You may be very familiar with the "healthy heart tick" for foods that are recognised as being good to keep our hearts healthy. So perhaps we should have a similar healthy brain food tick as well? Certainly that could make life a lot simpler when choosing what to put in the shopping trolley each week. The good news is that much of what is good for the heart is also good for the brain. So following a brain healthy diet is relatively easy, as it includes much of what we already know is good for us.

The eating plan that appears to be the most brain-healthy is the Mediterranean diet.

THE MEDITERRANEAN DIET

What does this diet include? Looking back on family holidays as a child in the Mediterranean, it conjures up memories of fresh fish from the market, large beef tomatoes, lots of salads, olives and generous servings of olive oil. Studies have indicated that following the Mediterranean diet can reduce our relative risk of developing Alzheimer's disease.

The diet is more than just fish, tomatoes and olive oil though; it also includes plenty of vegetables, legumes, fruits, cereals, and moderate alcohol, while remaining low in dairy, red meat and other saturated fats.

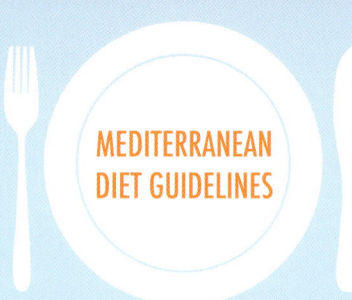

MEDITERRANEAN DIET GUIDELINES

Use olive oil in cooking and for dressings. Olive oil doesn't enjoy high heat; it burns. Avocado oil is a great alternative.

Eat more vegetables, especially green leafy vegetables and include some fruit and legumes.

Eat fish several times a week.

Reduce total red meat consumption. Choose white meat such as chicken as an alternative.

Use fresh produce whenever possible; make sauces using fresh tomato, garlic and onion.

Reduce consumption of dairy such as butter, cream, and processed foods including "fast foods," sweets, pastries and sugar-sweetened beverages.

Enjoy a moderate consumption of red wine, if you drink alcohol.

Drink lots of "aqua pura," i.e. water!

A study published in JAMA in 2009 looked at 1,875 people in New York who followed a Mediterranean-style diet. Of these people, 382 had mild cognitive impairment. Over the course of 4.5 years, a further 275 people in the group went on to develop cognitive impairment. It was found that those who had adhered most closely to the Mediterranean diet had a 28% lower relative risk of developing cognitive impairment compared to those who didn't.

Of those already diagnosed with cognitive impairment at the start of the study, again, those who adhered more closely to the Mediterranean diet were shown to be less likely to transition into full Alzheimer' disease. They showed a slower rate of cognitive decline, and were better able to maintain their normal activities of daily living, thereby continuing to enjoy a better quality of life as well as living longer.

The implications of this study suggest that following the Mediterranean diet may play an important role in reducing your risk of developing cognitive impairment by improving cholesterol levels, blood sugar levels, blood vessel health and reducing inflammation in the body.

The same group of researchers recently released further findings from MRI scans of the original subject group. Those who had most closely adhered to the Mediterranean diet showed fewer signs of brain damage in the form of brain infarcts. These are small areas of brain cell death, which can be associated with small vessel disease of the brain and contribute to vascular dementia.

New research from Spain has found that following the Mediterranean diet halved the incidence of new onset diabetes in a population, compared to those following a low-fat diet. This is particularly important, as diabetes is a known risk factor for dementia. Reducing the risk of diabetes through diet is a huge plus for maintaining better brain health.

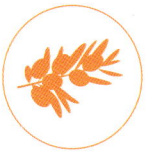

SMARTER THINKING: *Keeping to an eating plan similar to the Mediterranean diet based on leafy green vegetables, fish, olive oil, some red wine and less red meat and dairy will help maintain your brain health and reduce your risk of cognitive decline or dementia.*

GO FISH

Fish has to be the number one brain food. And not any old fish, either. Cold water, fatty fish is the best and includes such choices as wild salmon, tuna, mackerel, herring, sardines and anchovies, to name a few. These fish are full of Omega-3 fatty acids.

Fish on Fridays was a family ritual we adhered to in my childhood. Not for any religious association although it does have strong ties in some beliefs, but because it was Friday and that was the day we ate fish. Even at school (where we endured school dinners) we had fish on Fridays.

Eating fish is known to be good for our hearts as well as our brains.

And it would be great to have several Fridays each week because the recommendation from research is that we should be having two to three meals of fish per week.

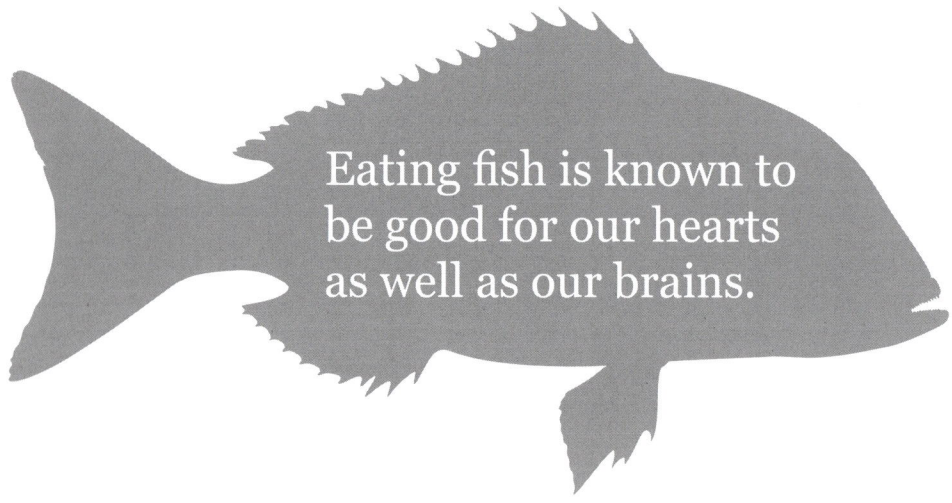

Eating fish is known to be good for our hearts as well as our brains.

THE BENEFITS OF OMEGA-3

The body cannot produce these essential fatty acids so we have to include them in our diet. Our brains are composed of 60% fat so it is essential we have a sufficient amount of the right sort of fatty acids to allow the brain to function normally.

When we eat fat, it is digested and broken down into fatty acid molecules. One of the main fats made by the brain is called docosahexaenoic acid (DHA). These molecules are then used by the body to assemble specialised fats used in every brain cell membrane to provide structure and functionality.

Myelin is a protective fatty sheath that enables our nerve fibres to conduct electrical messages much more quickly, and Omega-3s provide the essential building blocks.

Omega-3 fatty acids make prostaglandins, which are active substances involved in the brain. They regulate the release of neurotransmitters, the brain chemicals that brain cells use to send messages to each other. In the body, prostaglandins help to reduce blood pressure.

If we lack sufficient DHA then the brain cell membrane integrity is affected. This also tends to happen as we age. One of the outcomes from this is an increased risk of depression.

An imbalance of essential fatty acids has also been linked to hyperactivity, obsessive-compulsive disorder, bipolar disorder and schizophrenia. Here it is thought that having insufficient fatty acids in the brain cell membranes leads to the brain experiencing sensory overload.

Patients with Alzheimer's and Parkinson's disease have also displayed a loss of these fatty acids in their cell membranes.

Increasing dietary Omega-3 intake may have a protective effect against Parkinson's disease. In Parkinson's, the brain cells responsible for producing dopamine (a brain neurotransmitter associated with motor control), are greatly reduced. In laboratory studies, increasing Omega-3 in the diets of mice appeared to protect the brain from developing Parkinson's disease.

Nutritional studies in the elderly suggest that a diet sufficient in Omega-3s is vital to help maintain memory and cognition.

Eating fish has been shown in studies to help prevent stroke. In older, healthy people it also seems to reduce the number of silent brain infarcts, which can lead to stroke, dementia, and a loss of thinking skills. Vascular dementia (linked to stroke and high blood pressure) is the second most common form of dementia after Alzheimer's disease.

- In a study in Finland, brain scans of 3,660 people over the age of 65 were taken at five-year intervals. These people routinely ate fish three times a week. Their brain scans showed a 26% lower risk of brain infarcts simply by eating fish.

So what happens if you hate eating fish, or are allergic?

Fortunately we can get our Omega-3s from other sources including flax seed, walnuts, and green, leafy vegetables.

Of course it is possible to take fish oil capsules. It is preferable to look for wild fish oil capsules (which have a higher potency of Omega-3s). Taking one to two capsules a day is a great start to ensure your diet gets enough of those helpful Omega-3s.

OMEGA-3 FATTY ACID CONTENT OF FISH AND OTHER FOOD

The recommended daily amount of Omega-3 fatty acids from fish is 200–600 mg and from plants it is 1–2 g.

The following list from the Smart Food Centre and Graduate School of Medicine, University of Wollongong, details the approximate amounts of Omega-3 fatty acids per 60 g serving of varieties of fish:

SARDINES		**1,500mg**
SALMON (FRESH ATLANTIC)		**1,200mg**
SMOKED SALMON		**1,000mg**
CANNED SALMON		**500mg**
TROUT (FRESH RAINBOW)		**350mg**
GEM FISH		**300mg**
BLUE-EYE TREVALLA		**250mg**
SHARK (FLAKE)		**250mg**
SQUID		**250mg**
SCALLOP		**200mg**

CALAMARI ....▶ **200mg**

ABALONE ....▶ **170mg**

SEA MULLET ....▶ **170mg**

CANNED TUNA ....▶ **145mg**

ORANGE ROUGHY OR SEA PERCH ....▶ **7mg**

The following are approximate amounts of Omega-3 fatty acids per 60g serving of other foods:

TWO SLICES OF FISH OIL-ENRICHED WHITE BREAD ....▶ **27mg**

LEAN BEEF OR LAMB ....▶ **40mg**

ONE FISH OIL-ENRICHED EGG ....▶ **200mg**

FISH OIL-ENRICHED MARGARINE (10G) ....▶ **60mg**

ONE REGULAR EGG ....▶ **40mg**

A WORD OF CAUTION ON MERCURY

While it is recommended to eat two or more fish meals a week, it is wise to avoid fish that are high in mercury. Excess mercury appears to affect the nervous system, causing: numb or tingling fingers, lips and toes; developmental delays in walking and talking in children; muscle and joint pain; and increased risk of heart attack.

You may have heard about the concerns raised about the amount of mercury found in fish. Mercury is a neurotoxin; it can cause damage to the brain and central nervous system and is of particular concern in pregnancy and in babies and young children whose brains are not fully developed.

We can't avoid mercury in fish. Mercury is a naturally occurring element. It is also a by-product from some industrial processes and is released into the environment. In water, micro-organisms consume the mercury, transforming it into a more dangerous form called methylmercury. Small fish eat these organisms and the mercury accumulates in their flesh and skin. Bigger fish eat the smaller fish. The potential is for the biggest, longest-living fish such as shark, swordfish and tuna to accumulate the highest levels of mercury, which we then eat.

But despite these concerns, it appears that the benefits outweigh the risks overall. An article published in the Journal of the American Medical Association (JAMA) in 2006 calculated that the risk for 100,000 people eating farmed salmon twice a week for seventy years would lead to an additional 24 deaths from cancer. However, the consumption of the Omega-3s in that fish would prevent more than 7,000 deaths from heart disease.

Current recommendations include fish two to three times a week in our diet. Those considered more at risk from the effects of mercury (i.e., pregnant women, young babies and children), are recommended to eat fish less often, particularly fish such as shark, swordfish and tuna, but not to eliminate fish from your diet entirely.

SMARTER THINKING: Omega-3s are an essential component of a brain-healthy diet. Fish provides us with the highest concentration of these. Enjoy fish two to three times a week to gain the benefits of supporting our brains' structural integrity and function, and keep our brain cells firing at their best.

BERRIES

Blueberries, or "brain berries" as Dr. Steven Pratt has called them, have long been associated with having strong antioxidant and anti-inflammatory properties. This is largely due to the polyphenols (chemical substances found in many plants that act as antioxidants and provide colour to many fruits and vegetables) they contain. Anthocyanin is one, which gives the fruit their wonderful deep blue colour.

So can blueberries help your memory?

The earliest work suggesting blueberries could make a difference to memory was based on rat studies. Adding blueberry extract to the diet of ageing rats showed an increase in the learning capacity and motor skills in the rats, making them, essentially, mentally younger. Blueberry extract was shown to protect brain cells against atrophy by preserving the brain cell branches or dendrites and promoting new brain cell connections.

 **BLUEBERRIES COULD MAKE A DIFFERENCE TO MEMORY**

One human study published in early 2010 showed that drinking 2 to 2 1/2 cups of blueberry juice per day helped learning and memory in a group of 70-year-olds with early memory impairment. It's thought that the anthocyanin works in the hippocampus by activating specific proteins, which stimulate memory, improve neuronal or brain cell connections, neuronal communication and stimulate brain cell regeneration.

A U.K.-based study had previously shown that eating blueberries every day for 12 weeks produced an increase in spatial working memory during the period of the study. Remember too, it's not just blueberries that are good for your brain. All the deeply pigmented blue and red berries are super antioxidants as well. So include some strawberries, raspberries, blackberries and boysenberries daily.

RICH FRUITS

Food researchers have looked at the antioxidant properties of some Australian native fruits that have been enjoyed by the Aboriginal people for thousands of years. What they found is that some of these fruits have even higher antioxidant levels than blueberries, which may help encourage growers to continue to cultivate them. Some of those studies included the Kakadu plum, Illawarra plum, Burdekin plum, Davison's plum, riberry, red and yellow finger limes, Tasmanian pepper, brush cherry, Cedar Bay cherry muntries and the Molucca raspberry.

You may have noticed that many of the above are types of plum. Other research has compared 100 varieties of plums, peaches and nectarines and found many of these also contained high levels of antioxidants and phyto- nutrients to give blueberries a run for their money. The findings are encouraging as it means that we can all enjoy the potential health benefits from a wide range of fruit in our diets. The other bonus is that plums, for example, are relatively inexpensive compared to blueberries. (And plums are often more portable when you're on the go.)

And yes, there is more. Apart from having a high level of antioxidants and polyphenols, blueberries exert an anti-inflammatory effect on the brain. A U.S. researcher found that feeding rats a 2% blueberry extract (equivalent to humans enjoying a ½ cup of blueberries) was neuroprotective in preserving brain cell dendrites and synapses, effectively protecting the brain from atrophy and memory loss. These findings are encouraging and hopefully will be reproduced in humans.

 **SMARTER THINKING:** *Eating fruit, especially the deeply pigmented blue and red berries and plums, provides our brains with powerful antioxidants that have been shown in studies to support our brains' ability to learn and remember better. They are readily available, portable and yummy to eat.*

CHOCOLATE: MY FAVOURITE BRAIN FOOD

Mmm, chocolate. I really enjoy eating good chocolate as a treat. How boring life would be without being able to savour some really good quality chocolate from time to time.

And it would appear I am not alone. Australians as a nation rank ninth in the world for consumption of chocolate, with each of us eating on average six kilograms each year. (Don't feel guilty; the Swiss eat 10 kg per head!)

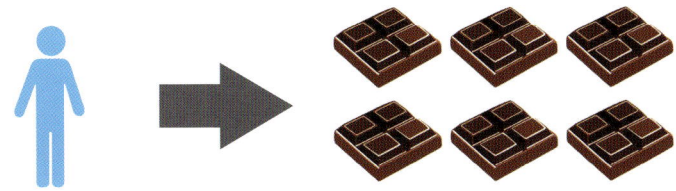

AUSTRALIANS CONSUME ON AVERAGE 6KG OF CHOCOLATE EACH YEAR

So, having consumed those 30,500 calories, 1750 g of fat, 1270 g of cholesterol, 4950 g sodium, 3550 g of carbohydrates and 540 g of protein, should we be concerned with our health as a result?

DOES CHOCOLATE CONTRIBUTE TO DISEASE?

The results of a study from Harvard reported that men over the age of 65 who ate chocolate several times a month actually lived longer than those who overindulged or denied themselves any chocolate at all.

So, it would appear that abstinence is actually worse than enjoying some chocolate occasionally!

And let's get rid of the acne myth. Chocolate has absolutely no bearing on acne at all. Even though your mother may have told you eating chocolate would give you pimples, it's not true. However, eating a healthy diet with lots of fruit and vegetables and some chocolate would be the best way to go to keep your skin glowing and healthy.

Eating too much of anything, including chocolate, a high calorie food, can contribute to weight gain. Being overweight or obese is not good for your general health and will predispose you to diabetes, which is definitely not good for your brain. So, moderation is the key.

Chocolate is best enjoyed as a small (e.g. 40 grams) regular treat. Do make sure it is good quality chocolate, and preferably dark.

SHOULD CHOCOLATE BE EATEN FOR HEALTH BENEFITS AND IS IT GOOD FOR OUR BRAIN?

Real or "dark" chocolate is packed full of goodies.

Over three hundred active substances have been identified in chocolate.

It contains some important minerals such as magnesium, phosphorous, potassium and iron as well as antioxidants including vitamins A1, B1, C, D and E. It's been suggested that one reason why women crave chocolate pre-menstrually is for the magnesium it contains. Whether or not that is true, it sounds like a reasonable explanation to give when that family bar of chocolate has disappeared.

Unfortunately not all chocolate is good for us. White chocolate is actually not chocolate at all; it contains cacao butter and sugar, but no cacao solids. Milk chocolate contains milk, as its name suggests, but lacks the flavonol content that provides the health benefits.

FLAVONOLS AND DARK CHOCOLATE

Cocoa, or chocolate, contains powerful antioxidants called flavonols or phenols. Dark chocolate contains the highest concentration of these. (They are also found in blueberries, green tea and red wine.) Studies have recently shown some potential benefits on blood pressure, as well as providing an energy boost and an anxiolytic effect so we feel less stressed.

Sunil Kocher at the Nestlé Research Centre in Switzerland (sounds a great place to work!) did a study on 30 stressed men and women where they consumed 40 g of dark chocolate a day for 14 days. He measured their stress hormones and the results indicated that eating chocolate helped to modulate their stress levels.

I could have told him that. Doesn't everyone eat extra chocolate when feeling stressed?

A study in the U.K. by Professor Ian McDonald from Nottingham University used a particularly concentrated flavonol cocoa drink that they formulated especially for the study. The drink caused increased cerebral blood flow (for a couple of hours) to key areas of the brain in subjects. The researchers suggested the increased blood flow and hence oxygen supply to the brain could be associated with increased brain performance in specific tasks and a boost to general alertness. Though how much

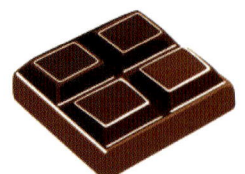

COCOA, OR CHOCOLATE, CONTAINS POWERFUL ANTIOXIDANTS CALLED FLAVONOLS OR PHENOLS. DARK CHOCOLATE CONTAINS THE HIGHEST CONCENTRATION OF THESE.

commercially available chocolate one would have to eat to produce this effect is unknown.

Chocolate has been investigated for its role of protecting against stroke. A Canadian study of over 44,000 people showed that eating one serving (size not known) of chocolate a week was associated with a 22% reduction in risk of stroke. In a second study of over 1,000 people, those who ate 50 grams of chocolate a week had a 46% reduction in the risk of dying from a stroke compared to those who didn't eat any.

A population of Kuna Indians who live on islands close to Panama have been found to experience virtually no problems with elevated blood pressure or cardiovascular disease. This has been attributed to a popular local beverage of very bitter cocoa they consume in large quantities – up to five cups each day – as well as incorporating it in their diet. It's very high in the flavonoid epicatechin. The epicatechin itself appears to promote natural pathways for the body to protect itself from free radical damage by helping the body to process nitric oxide, which is essential for healthy blood vessels and hence also helps to regulate blood pressure.

Different chocolate contains different amounts of bioactive epicatechin and much is

Several studies have shown that chocolate can produce a modest reduction in systolic blood pressure in hypertensive patients.

destroyed in the commercial production of chocolate. So just because it may call itself dark chocolate, it doesn't mean it is always good for you.

Several studies have shown that chocolate can produce a modest reduction in systolic blood pressure in hypertensive patients. It had no effect in people who were normotensive. The flavonoids in the chocolate increase the formation of nitric oxide in the blood vessel walls, helping blood vessels to dilate and, as a result, lower the blood pressure.

WHY DOES EATING CHOCOLATE MAKE US FEEL GOOD?

Chocolate contains a number of bioactive compounds including caffeine, theobromine and phenylethylamine that are associated with stimulating brain chemical or neurotransmitter production and keeps us alert. It contains tryptophan – an essential amino acid that the body uses to produce serotonin, our "happy" neurotransmitter. Having a higher level of serotonin helps us to feel good and less anxious.

Another chemical found in chocolate is anandamide (meaning "bliss" in Sanskrit). This is a neurotransmitter also produced by the brain and is a natural brain stimulant.

Two other chocolate chemicals work to slow down our body's ability to break down the anandamide. Anandamide works on the brain receptors associated with the release of the neurotransmitter dopamine, which is associated with a feeling of well-being.

But the main reason eating chocolate makes us feel so good is thought to be the endorphins it releases that stimulate the brain. There is now research to support that eating a small (around 40 g) amount of good quality dark chocolate may be good for our hearts and brains. So now we don't have to feel too guilty about indulging a little bit!

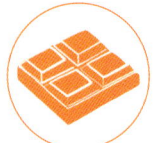

SMARTER THINKING: *There are some suggested brain benefits of eating chocolate. As with all things, just because having some is good for you, it doesn't mean having lots is better. Eating a lot of chocolate adds a significant calorie, sugar and fat burden, which could be of substantial detriment to our health.*

DRINKING RED WINE

A little bit of what you fancy can do you good in relation to enjoying a glass or two of red wine. As with many things though, it is a question of moderation in order to get the benefits. Overdoing it can have a negative outcome.

Drinking red wine has been touted for its health benefits for some time, yet it is only relatively recently that indulging in a taste of one's favourite Shiraz, Cabernet Sauvignon or Pinot noir was found to be of benefit for our brain health.

It is well known that overindulging in any form of alcohol can lead to loss of social inhibitions, poor judgement and a bad headache the next day.

Binge drinking continues to be a major heath concern particularly amongst the young. Alcoholism takes a terrible toll not only on the person affected but also on their family and friends.

Yet a small amount of alcohol is now thought to be good for our health in a number of ways.

A long term study of over 12,500 women showed that those who enjoyed one drink a day on average scored higher on tests of mental clarity than non-drinkers. Another study published in the Journal of the American Medical Association (JAMA) showed that people who drank between one and six drinks a week had a 50% reduction in their risk of dementia and heart disease.

RISK OF DEVELOPING DEMENTIA

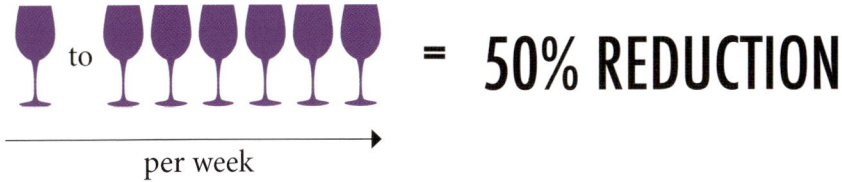

to ... per week = **50% REDUCTION**

However, having more than two drinks a day increased the risk of dementia by 22%. Alcohol-related dementia is a known, major cause of memory impairment.

As you get older your tolerance for alcohol diminishes, your body takes longer to detoxify the body from the alcohol, meaning there is greater potential for the alcohol to do damage.

Alcohol itself is a poison and damages brain cells. It is associated with an increased risk of breast cancer in women, colon cancer and liver damage.

In alcohol-related dementia, damage to the brain leads to memory impairment and learning difficulties. Nutritional deficiencies including B1 or thiamine can also develop, contributing to both poor brain cell and nerve health.

Other issues associated with alcohol-related dementia include:

- Problems with short-term memory
- Personality change
- Difficulty with logical thinking (planning, organising and judgement)
- Poor social skills
- Balance problems
- Decreased initiative

This type of dementia is most common in men aged 45 to 65 who have a long history of alcohol abuse. Women can, of course, also be affected.

The important thing here is that the dementia associated with alcohol will not progress if the person can stop drinking and correct any nutritional deficiencies.

The important thing here is that the dementia associated with alcohol will not progress if the person can stop drinking and correct any nutritional deficiencies.

The double-edged sword of alcohol is that, conversely, moderate alcohol intake has been shown in a study to confer long-term cognitive protection and reduce the risk of dementia in middle-aged and older adults.

Of 3,069 people over the age of 75 years who were moderate drinkers (eight to 14 drinks per week) over a six-year period, saw a 37% risk reduction of dementia compared to non-drinkers.

However, the protection is lost if cognitive impairment is already present. Any consumption of alcohol by a person with cognitive impairment will be associated with a faster rate of decline, especially if they were in the healthy drinking sector (less than 14 drinks per week).

WHAT'S IN WINE THAT MAKES IT BENEFICIAL?

Researchers have been focussing their attention on resveratrol, the antioxidant found in red wine. Oxidation is a normal chemical reaction that takes place in the body. It results in the production of free radicals, which can lead to cell damage. Antioxidants work to prevent or slow the oxidative process. Resveratrol is also found in a number of other plant sources. It was first isolated from white hellebore roots and Japanese knotweed. In addition to grapes, it is also found in peanuts, mulberries, blueberries, lily, spruce, and the extensive eucalypt family (over 400 different species).

RED WINE OR WHITE?

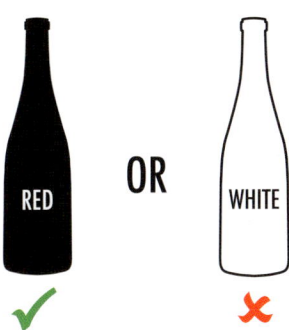

The question often asked is whether it is better to drink red wine or white wine. The answer is red because the grape skins contain the highest amount of resveratrol. In red wine production, the grapes and skins are crushed and left to ferment together for a longer period of time, whereas in white wine production, the skins are removed early on in the process. The varieties of grape with the highest levels of resveratrol found so far are Labrusca, Muscadine and Vitis Vinifera.

In England, current studies are underway to test resveratrol levels in different red wines, with the idea that one day we may buy a bottle of red wine not just based on the grape variety or label, but rather on its beneficial resveratrol content.

Red wine has been linked to the French Paradox, where the high level of red wine consumption appears to protect the French population against heart disease that's normally associated with a high fat diet. Resveratrol has been shown to be cardio-protective and may have potential therapeutic effects in cancer management, as well as being useful to prevent diabetes, inflammation and dementia.

It is now believed that inflammation plays a role in the development of Alzheimer's disease.

HOW DOES IT WORK?

It is now believed that inflammation plays a role in the development of Alzheimer's disease. In the Framingham Heart Study, those people identified with the highest levels of cytokines (inflammation markers) in their blood were likely to have an increased risk of developing Alzheimer's disease.

Resveratrol does not appear to have any effect itself in preventing the build-up of beta amyloid plaques in the brain, but it does stimulate their removal. This is an indirect effect of the resveratrol stimulating the body's own protoeasomes, which are cellular protein disposal units that grab hold and dispose of the beta amyloid.

This is thought to be the mechanism by which resveratrol exerts its neuroprotective effect.

Resveratrol has also been shown in other studies to stimulate the production of neuroprotective enzymes such as haem-oxidase.

The interest in resveratrol has stimulated a burgeoning new industry keen to produce resveratrol in supplement form. However it remains unclear as to what the ideal dosage would be, and some researchers have urged caution.

SMARTER THINKING: *Alcohol is a neurotoxin. However, some studies indicate that drinking a small amount of red wine can be of benefit to the brain from the resveratrol it contains. This is not a reason to start drinking alcohol. Resveratrol is available in other foods and in supplement form without the additional negative risk of alcohol.*

CAFFEINE AND COFFEE DRINKING

How many of us look forward to that first cup of coffee or tea in the morning just to get going? Apparently 90% of Americans rely on that first cup of coffee.

Caffeine has been described as the world's most widely-consumed psychostimulant. We like our caffeine shot because we believe it gives us that mental edge, so we are more alert and firing on all cylinders. But does it really give us the edge we think it does?

Whether it be in our tea, coffee, cola or energy drink, the caffeine will certainly make us more alert because it is a stimulant.

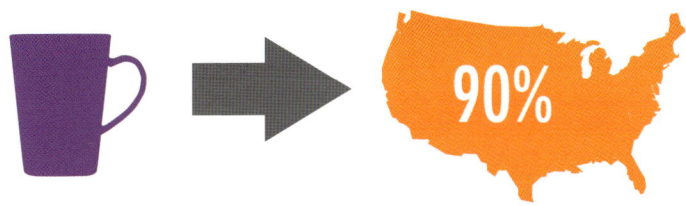

REPORTS SUGGEST 90% OF AMERICANS RELY ON A CUP OF COFFEEE TO KICK START THEIR DAY

HOW DOES CAFFEINE AFFECT THE BRAIN?

When we drink our caffeine beverage the caffeine competes with a naturally occurring chemical called adenosine, which gradually accumulates during the day and normally has a slowing-down effect on our brain cells, helping prepare us to go to sleep. By blocking the effect of the adenosine, the caffeine causes the rate of brain cells firing to speed up.

This increased brain activity and neuronal firing rate is detected by the pituitary gland in the brain and interprets this as a possible red alert. The fight-or-flight response is initiated and adrenaline is pumped from adrenal glands through the body, ready to help us avoid any perceived danger.

Once the effect of the caffeine starts to wear off, we are likely to feel more fatigued from all that extra brain activity required to keep us alert. So we look to that next cup of coffee, and the cycle is repeated.

In general terms, sadly, this increased mental alertness is not accompanied by increased mental performance. Drinking too much coffee leaves us tired.

Detoxing from caffeine is well known for the nasty headache it can produce. This is due to the blood vessels in the brain constricting when no caffeine is around. Caffeine causes them to dilate. The first few days of withdrawal can also be associated with general aches and pains, extreme tiredness and even a feeling of depression. By day six or seven however, the body will have recovered, your level of anxiety will have subsided, your blood pressure will be lower, your sleep pattern will have improved and mentally you will be functioning just as well as when you were drinking coffee.

Many of us know that drinking coffee late at night can keep us awake. Peak plasma levels are reached in 40 to 50 minutes after drinking coffee. But the half-life of caffeine is about six hours. If you know you are sensitive to caffeine's effects then remember that having a cup of coffee at 4 p.m. is going to keep you awake when you want to go to sleep at 10 p.m., as you will still have 50% of the caffeine in your system.

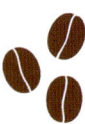 # CAFFEINE BOOSTS DOPAMINE LEVELS

Some good news about caffeine is that it boosts dopamine levels. Dopamine is an important neurotransmitter that helps regulate mood. Having more dopamine heightens your feel-good factor.

Maybe that's why so many of us really enjoy our coffee; it makes us feel good. But too much caffeine increases our level of anxiety and makes us jittery.

SO ARE THERE ANY BENEFITS OF CAFFEINE FOR THE BRAIN?

There has been an enormous amount of research done looking at caffeine and the brain. The results indicate that caffeine does have a number of beneficial effects in normalising brain function and acting as a neuroprotective agent.

It has been shown to help reduce beta amyloid plaques. Caffeine promotes increased neuronal firing and that is thought to be what helps to increase short-term memory skills and reaction times.

Some epidemiological studies have indicated a neuroprotective effect in Parkinson's disease.

A study carried out in Finland found caffeine consumption of three to five cups a day was associated with a lower risk of dementia compared to those who drank either no coffee or only one or two cups a day. A separate study showed that older French women over the age of 65 who drank three cups of coffee a day had improved word recall and improved brain power.

And finally, animal studies have shown that caffeine can protect the brain from the damaging effects of excess cholesterol.

SO HOW MUCH CAFFEINE IS GOOD FOR US?

Depending on your body size and particular tolerance levels, an average person should probably stay within 300 to 400 mg a day.

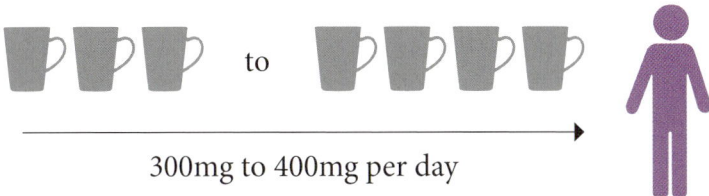

300mg to 400mg per day

Approx. Serving   **Caffeine content***

COFFEE (1 CUP/250ML) ....➤ **72 – 130 mg**

TEA (1 CUP/250ML) ....➤ **20 – 90 mg**

COLA DRINK (350ML) ....➤ **30 mg**

ESPRESSO (1 DEMI-CUP/30ML) ....➤ **58 – 76 mg**

RED BULL (250ML) ....➤ **80 mg**

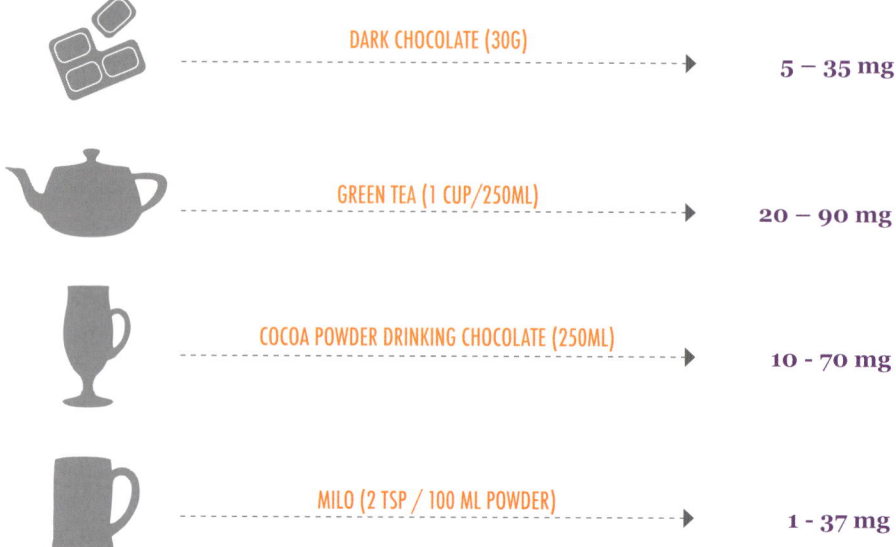

DARK CHOCOLATE (30G)   5 – 35 mg

GREEN TEA (1 CUP/250ML)   20 – 90 mg

COCOA POWDER DRINKING CHOCOLATE (250ML)   10 - 70 mg

MILO (2 TSP / 100 ML POWDER)   1 - 37 mg

* The caffeine contents indicated above vary greatly as a function of food quality and processing

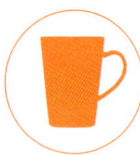

SMARTER THINKING: *Coffee will certainly help to keep you awake and alert; just don't expect it to make any difference to your mental performance. Excess caffeine can cause insomnia, agitation and restlessness, so keep your intake of daily caffeine to a safe level for your body and brain.*

TURMERIC

I was having a conversation with a group of ladies recently. The topic of conversation was the use of supplements and natural herbs and spices that are supposed to be good for our brains. One lady advised me that every morning she pours a good dollop of flaxseed oil onto her breakfast cereal along with some linseed, sunflower and almond mix (LSA), psyllium and a heaped teaspoon of turmeric.

I obviously looked a bit surprised at her choice of spice to zing up her cereal as she then went on to tell me she had got quite used to the taste and didn't mind it. Personally I yet remain to be convinced about the flavour combination. So, what is the deal with turmeric and why would this person be so keen to be adding it to her breakfast?

Turmeric or Curcuma longa is an Indian spice and a member of the ginger family. It has a wonderful yellow hue that lends its colour to curry, mustard and piccalilli relish.

Some years ago it was reported that the Indian subcontinent enjoyed a significantly lower incidence of dementia or Alzheimer's in its population compared to Western societies. One study in rural North India reported an incidence of 0.62% in those over the age of 55 years and 1.07% in those aged 65 and older. Compare that to 10% for 65-year-olds in the Western world. There have been a number of reasons postulated as to why this should be. One of the thoughts put forward is that it is due to the curcumin found in turmeric, which is consumed in vast quantities every day in curries.

The curcuminoids in the turmeric have been associated with a number of significant health benefits and several studies have been completed looking at how it may afford protection against neuro-degenerative disease.

LET'S HAVE A LOOK AT THE RESEARCH

One of the hallmark findings in Alzheimer's disease is plaque in the brain made of a substance called beta amyloid. The body has its own defence system in the form of scavenging cells called macrophages to try and get rid of this plaque. These cells travel around the brain trying to remove any amyloid they find. One study looked at the effect of treating these macrophages with curcumin and found that the macrophages were better able to gobble up the beta amyloid with an improvement rate of 50%.

Curcumin has potent anti-inflammatory and anti-oxidant effects. Because it is thought that inflammation plays a role in the development of Alzheimer's, studies were done to see whether anti-inflammatory drugs, and/or curcumin (with its anti-inflammatory effect), could be useful in treating beta amyloid plaque build-up.

One study conducted at UCLA looked at the anti-inflammatory effect of curcumin versus ibuprofen (a commonly used anti-inflammatory drug). Using rats with beta amyloid in their brains, separately the curcumin and the ibuprofen were shown to provide equivalent protection from the inflammatory damage caused by the beta amyloid. The curcumin reduced the amount of plaque in the rat brains by up to 80% at low dose, and the rats given the curcumin performed better on spatial memory tests compared to the control group. Curcumin is one of the few compounds that can cross the blood brain barrier and is able to bind to amyloid protein fragments, which are then unable to clump together to form plaques.

There was initially great excitement that the anti-inflammatories could be a useful therapeutic tool in treating Alzheimer's disease. Sadly, follow-up clinical trials in human patients with Alzheimer's disease who were prescribed anti-inflammatory drugs such as ibuprofen, only produced limited or negative results. Likewise the Alzheimer's Disease Anti-inflammatory Prevention Trial (ADAPT) cognitive function tests using another commonly prescribed anti-inflammatory, Naprosyn, similarly showed no benefit in improving cognitive function in older adults. A glimmer of hope remains to examine whether there is a possibility that taking the non-steroidal anti-inflammatory drugs (NSAID) prior to the clinical onset of any cognitive decline could be useful. This has yet to be shown.

HOW DOES THE CURCUMIN EXERT ITS EFFECT?

Dr. A. Ramamoorthy at the University of Michigan has shown that the curcumin inserts itself into cell membranes, changing the physical properties of the membrane rather than interacting directly with the membrane proteins.

He is now working on determining the relative potency of a variety of curcuminoid derivatives that could potentially lead to new compounds being formulated as treatments. He is also investigating how curcumin exerts its effects on the formation of beta amyloid.

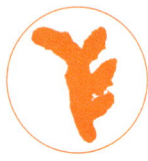

SMARTER THINKING: So if eating curry with turmeric may assist in keeping our minds sharp as we age, how much should we be eating? Dr. Sally Frautschy, Associate Professor at UCLA, who eats curry four times a week, suggests one tablespoon or 200 mg per day. (But I think I still prefer to eat my turmeric in curry rather than on my breakfast cereal.)

EGGS

There used to be an advert telling us to "go to work on an egg." Cute slogan notwithstanding, recently people have become wary of eggs because of salmonella scares and the belief eggs contain too much cholesterol.

It's come to light now that the amount of cholesterol in the egg yolk is really of little significance to how it affects your body's levels of cholesterol. So good news, we are now being encouraged to enjoy eggs again, even as many as six per week.

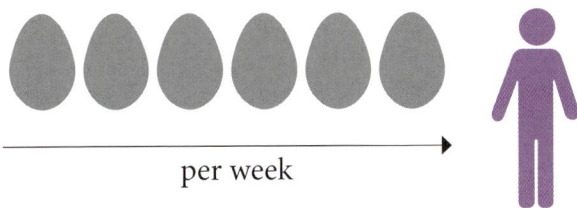

per week

Eggs are a fantastic source of lean protein. They are also a rich source of choline, which is found in sardines, liver, soya beans, lecithin and peanuts as well.

Choline is an essential nutrient we need to form acetylcholine, a crucial brain chemical or neurotransmitter. We need choline in our diets because the body cannot produce enough of the amount required by our brains and bodies. It is the egg yolk that provides the richest source of choline, 200 mg per yolk. Adult women need approximately 425 mg choline per day. Men need 550 mg.

Choline is essential for good brain health:

APPROXIMATE CHOLINE PER DAY

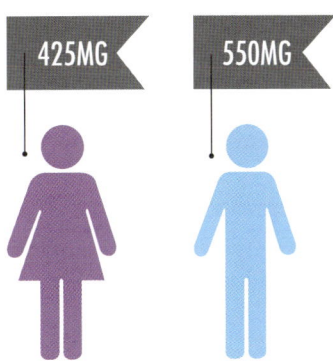

- Combined with other vitamins, it helps to form acetylcholine that is key for encoding memory. Acetylcholine is also essential for muscle control.

- Choline helps to boost levels of dopamine and other brain neurotransmitters such as citicholine. Having adequate dopamine assists our assertiveness and motivation, autonomic system and immune function.

- It is an essential component of brain cell membranes, vital for their integrity and plasticity. It is used to produce phospholipids, phosphatidylcholine and sphingomyelin, which are found in all of our cell membranes and make up much of the brain.

- Choline is vital to healthy brain development in the unborn child and in early childhood, and to maintain good memory throughout life.

- A lack of choline can lead to deficiency of folic acid, a B vitamin that is also crucial for brain health.

- Choline and its derivative, betaine, are associated with reducing homocysteine. Homocysteine is a normal by-product of metabolism but in excess is linked to increased inflammatory responses, potentially causing heart disease and dementia.

Some studies have suggested that supplementing our diets with choline can have beneficial effects on memory. Choline given to pregnant rats resulted in their offspring having superior learning ability and better memory recall, the effect being seen throughout their lifespan. This effect has not been shown in humans.

Other studies have not been able to say clearly whether supplementing choline in later life is of benefit to improving memory. It is recognised that the body's ability to absorb choline diminishes as we get older.

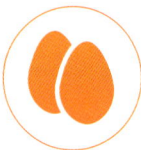

SMARTER THINKING: There are lots of other good reasons to enjoy eggs, but for boosting choline levels and helping to maintain a healthy brain, enjoying six free-range eggs a week is a great start. So as they like to say, "get cracking."

WATER

Water is essential to life. Our bodies are composed of over 70% water, and the brain alone comprises 85% water. So it is no wonder that in order to enjoy having our brains in optimum health we need to keep well hydrated.

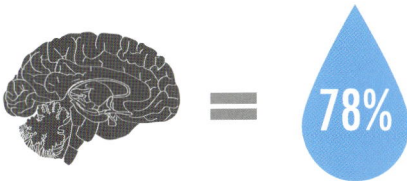

If you have ever been dehydrated or have seen someone who is, you will already know the serious effect it can have on one's body even at relatively low rates of dehydration.

Dehydration can lead to a number of symptoms including:

- Headache
- Dizziness
- Loss of concentration
- Lack of energy
- Dry skin
- Increased body temperature
- Constipation
- Pungent, darkly coloured urine

Cognitive performance is adversely affected even at low levels of two per cent dehydration and less. Neurons store water in vacuoles within the cells. With insufficient water, the neurons shrink and cellular communication slows down. The body's blood volume drops and our brains become at risk of overheating.

You may notice that your brain's processing speed is slower, your short-term memory is impaired and it is harder to pay attention.

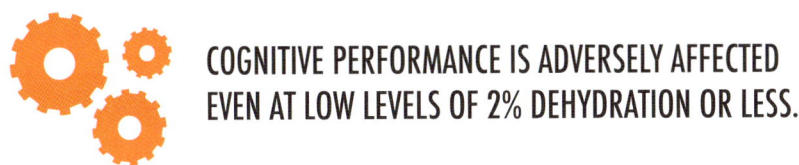

COGNITIVE PERFORMANCE IS ADVERSELY AFFECTED EVEN AT LOW LEVELS OF 2% DEHYDRATION OR LESS.

HOW MUCH WATER DO WE NEED?

Well, the old adage of six to eight glasses a day is about right. This is 1½ to 2 litres per day. It will vary according to body weight and activity. Heat exposure or vigorous exercise will also increase the amount needed.

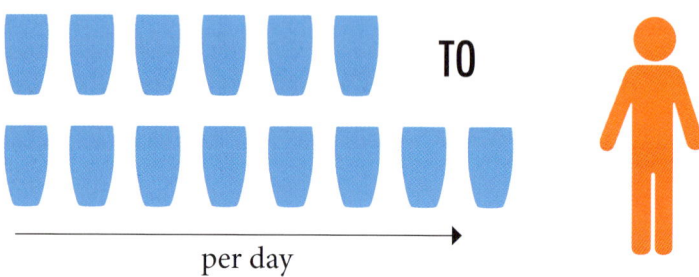

TO

per day

Excessive sweating from heat or exercise can result in fluid loss of several litres of body fluid per hour. When rehydrating, the body is capable of absorbing one litre of hour.

So it is recommended we drink water before, during and after exercise.

Thirst is an unreliable indicator of hydration. By the time we experience thirst we are likely to already be significantly dehydrated by two per cent.

The easiest way to check your level of hydration is to have a look at the colour of your urine. Ideally, it should be virtually clear. Darker shades of yellow or even brown indicate you are dehydrated and need to top up your water intake.

If you take vitamin supplements though, this can be misleading as the B vitamins in particular make urine go a rather beautiful, vivid yellow.

It is possible to overdo it and over-hydration with water is as much of a medical problem as dehydration. It can cause serious sodium imbalance and can lead to collapse, so care is required especially when rehydrating after exercise.

Having said that, most of us would benefit from increasing our water consumption. The bottled water industry pumps out billions of dollars' worth of (sometimes very expensive) water. Tap water is fine, although if you have a filter this can sometimes make the water taste better.

Children and the elderly are particularly at risk of dehydration.

Kids who are dehydrated will show a drop in cognitive and academic performance. This is surely a very good reason to ensure all children have adequate access to clean drinking water at school.

As we age, our ability to recognise thirst diminishes. A special area in the brain called the mid-cingulate cortex functions less well, making it harder to accurately gauge our level of thirst. This is why dehydration in the elderly is a common and significant problem.

Easy ways to increase your water consumption:

- Start your day with a glass of water as soon as you get out of bed.

- Drink a glass before you pour your first cup of coffee or tea.

- Have water on your desk at work and, for children, at school.

- Never pass a water fountain without stopping for a drink.

- Rather than reaching for a second cup of coffee or tea, drink water.

- When the waiter pours water at a restaurant, actually drink it.

Not everything that is wet or liquid is necessarily good for us in terms of hydration. Alcohol and caffeinated drinks are all dehydrators. Fruit juices do not quench thirst and contain lots of natural and sometimes artificial sugars. All those bottles of water with added nutrients are very expensive ways to drink water that would be better obtained from the tap or filter. Carbonated drinks are full of either sugar and/or additives and are not good nutrients at all, so are best completely avoided.

SMARTER THINKING: *Water is essential to maintain brain cell hydration and keep your brain working at its best. Next time you feel your energy fading, check first you are not simply dehydrated, and drink a glass of water. Thirst is a late message telling us to we need to drink more.*

THE ROLE OF HOMOCYSTEINE AND THE B VITAMINS

I often get asked about vitamin supplements for better brain health. There have been a lot of contradictory reports. Currently, other than taking a good quality multivitamin, there is probably little to commend in taking other supplements at this stage. However, a caveat on that relates to the B vitamins and their role in regulating an important amino acid in the body called homocysteine.

As previously in discussed in the Mediterranean diet, the food we choose to eat is important in helping our brain cells function well and stay at their best. Many studies have examined the different micronutrients, i.e., the vitamins and minerals we eat, to see what impact (if any), they may have in helping us keep our brains healthy.

In 2010, a report was published in the U.K. on the findings of a research study looking at the effect of the B vitamins on brain shrinkage. This was a small trial in Oxford to determine if administering large doses of B vitamins would lower blood homocysteine levels and lessen brain atrophy or shrinkage in elderly subjects who already had mild cognitive impairment.

THE SHRINKING BRAIN

Our brains start to shrink from the time we are in our early twenties. Not by much, around 0.2% per year. But once we reach the age of 60, the rate of shrinkage starts to increase to 0.5% per year.

In mild cognitive impairment (MCI), a person is having problems with memory loss, language difficulty and other problems beyond those normally expected simply through ageing.

Around 16% of people over the age of 70 develop MCI and half of these people subsequently go on to develop Alzheimer's disease. MCI is seen as a precursor for Alzheimer's. In MCI, the rate of brain shrinkage increases to 1% and by the time Alzheimer's is diagnosed it is around 2.5% per year.

RATE OF BRAIN SHRINKAGE

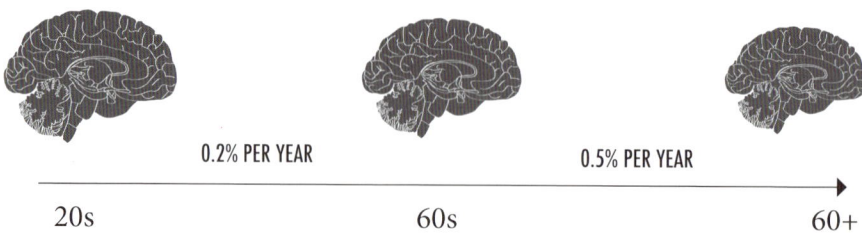

0.2% PER YEAR

0.5% PER YEAR

20s   60s   60+

WHAT IS HOMOCYSTEINE?

Homocysteine is an amino acid that is very important to the body's metabolism. It depends on the presence of folate, vitamin B6 and vitamin B12 (which we take in with our diet), to be kept to a normal range. In excess, homocysteine has been shown to be a risk factor for heart disease, brain atrophy, cognitive impairment and dementia.

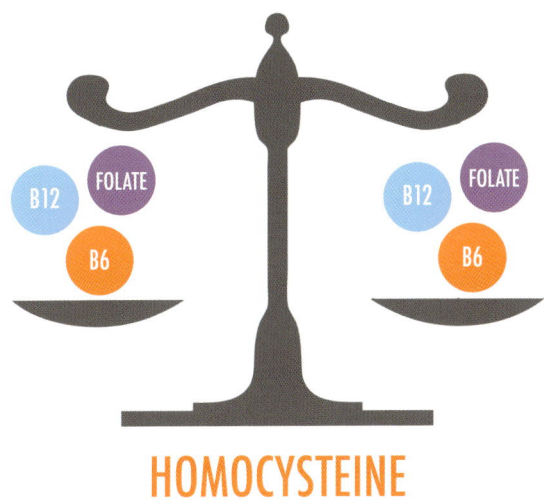

HOMOCYSTEINE

An elevated homocysteine level can double the risk of developing Alzheimer's disease. The findings came from part of the Framingham study that began in the 1960s. 1,500 women aged between 38 and 60 years completed a health questionnaire and had blood taken to determine homocysteine levels. Some 35 years later, the data was examined to see who within that group went on to develop Alzheimer's disease.

The results showed that having an elevated homocysteine level produced more than a doubling of the relative risk of developing Alzheimer's. It was associated with a 70% risk of developing any form of dementia. (As this study only looked at women, the results can't be extrapolated to men.)

What hasn't been determined either is whether the damage leading to the development of Alzheimer's disease or other forms of dementia is a result of the elevated homocysteine itself, or the associated vitamin deficiencies.

As we age, the incidence of folate and B12 deficiency tends to increase, as does the incidence of neurological disease. Animal studies have shown that folate, vitamin B12 and B6 deficiencies are linked to poorer memory and spatial learning and reduced blood supply to the hippocampus, the specialised brain area concerned with memory.

BIG DOSES OF VITAMIN B

In the Oxford trial, very large doses of B vitamins were used: 300 times the recommended daily intake (RDI) for vitamin B12, 15 times for Vitamin B6 and four times that for folic acid.

The co-author Helga Refsum from the University of Oslo stated that the vitamins were being used in the study as drugs, not as vitamin supplements. Because other research has not been done using similar high doses, it is unknown if using these megadoses will have any long-term effects. There have been studies elsewhere linking high-dose folate to an increased risk of cancer. Because of this, caution is advised against assuming that using high doses of vitamins is safe.

In the study, 168 people over the age of 70 with mild cognitive impairment were divided into two groups. One group received the mega dose vitamins and the other group received a placebo. MRI scans were used to measure brain volume at the beginning of the study and then annually over a two-year period.

The group taking the mega dose of vitamins showed an average reduction in the rate of brain atrophy of 30%. Moreover, those who had had the highest level of homocysteine at the beginning of the study showed the greatest reduction in shrinkage rate, by a massive 53%. Those who had received the vitamins also performed better overall on mental testing.

The inference from the study was that this may be a way to help reduce the number of people with mild cognitive impairment from progressing to full blown Alzheimer's.

The "how" of lowering homocysteine to produce this brain saving effect is not yet known.The results of such a small study, while encouraging, need to be followed up with a much larger study to verify the findings.

WHERE TO FROM HERE?

Science proves that B vitamins are important in helping us to maintain a normal nervous system.

We can obtain B vitamins from diet. Some foods are already fortified with B vitamins, especially folic acid. The role of folate in helping to prevent neural tube defects (spina bifida) in babies is well documented.

Good sources of B12 are found in fish, milk, meat, eggs and chicken.

Vitamin B6 is found in beans, meat, poultry, potatoes, bananas and tuna.

Folate (folic acid) is found in green leafy vegetables such as spinach and fortified breads and cereals.

Some foods are known to be rich in a substance called methionine. The body breaks down the methionine into homocysteine. So should we be avoiding those foods, and which ones are they?

Foods high in methionine include red meat, fish, beans, eggs, lentil, onions, yoghurt and seeds. But these foods are also good for us aren't they? Yes they are. The answer lies in the quality and balance of your diet. Eating foods high in methionine is not an issue when consumed as part of a balanced diet.

MODERATION IS THE SOLUTION

A mouse study from Temple University looked at how changing diet, even in early-to-moderate Alzheimer's disease, could make a difference in slowing down the rate of cognitive impairment. After feeding mice a high methionine diet, producing cognitive decline, this effect was then reversed by changing their diet to one that was low in methionine foods.

So we can enjoy a wide range of commonly eaten foods to provide us with a good intake of the B vitamins. A simple blood test can measure homocysteine levels and it is easy enough to take the B vitamins in supplement form. It just remains too early yet to recommend taking big doses to preserve our brains.

What is particularly encouraging from this study is that it may provide a simple and inexpensive treatment to reduce the number of people with MCI from progressing to full-blown Alzheimer's disease.

SMARTER THINKING: Eating a well-balanced diet to ensure you consume plenty of the essential vitamins and minerals, especially those foods which are high in the B group of vitamins helps to maintain a healthier brain.

WHAT IS VITAMIN D?

Vitamin D isn't really a vitamin as all. Your body produces vitamin D from ultraviolet exposure (UVB) to your skin. It actually functions more like a hormone in the body and has a wide variety of different and important functions. It promotes calcium absorption in the gut and helps maintain normal mineralisation of bones and bone growth.

It is also involved in your immune system, neuromuscular function, modulates cell growth and reduces inflammation.

Because of this, vitamin D has been extensively researched to try and better understand its various roles. Testing reveals that many people have either insufficient or an actual deficiency of vitamin D, which is associated with a number of diseases including rickets, certain cancers, diabetes and cardiovascular disease. Inadequate levels of vitamin D are a major public health concern worldwide. It is estimated that 31% of all Australian adults have inadequate levels of vitamin D, despite living in a country characterised by its high levels of sunshine.

Vitamin D is important to our brain health. Having too little vitamin D has been associated with:

- Poor balance
- Decreased muscle strength
- Low mood and depression
- Cognitive dysfunction

HOW MUCH TIME DO YOU NEED IN THE SUN?

That will vary according to skin type, amount of skin pigmentation, the time of year and latitude where you live. A rough estimate thought to be sufficient to prevent deficiency is between five to 15 minutes of sunlight exposure to your face and upper arms, between four to six days a week.

 A ROUGH ESTIMATE THOUGHT TO BE SUFFICIENT TO PREVENT DEFICIENCY IS BETWEEN FIVE TO 15 MINUTES OF SUNLIGHT EXPOSURE TO YOUR FACE AND UPPER ARMS, BETWEEN FOUR TO SIX DAYS A WEEK.

Because sunscreen of factor eight and above will prevent up to 95% of vitamin D conversion in the skin, the recommendation is for only short exposures to the sun without sunscreen outside the hours of 10 a.m. and 3 p.m.

In summer time you only need 10-15 minutes of sun exposure, and in winter, around 30 minutes.

HAS THE APPLICATION OF SUNSCREEN CONTRIBUTED TO THE EXTENSIVE INCIDENCE OF VITAMIN D DEFICIENCY?

It is too simplistic to say that sunscreen has led to such widespread vitamin D deficiency.

Many countries such as Finland that have relatively little sun exposure, and therefore less use for sunscreen, also have populations with significantly low or deficient vitamin D levels.

The risk to our health from sun cancers including melanoma is significant, so it's vital we all continue with the "Slip, Slop, Slap" campaign to cover up from the harmful effects of the sun. Melanoma is the deadliest form of skin cancer and is triggered by UVA (long UV wavelengths). Vitamin D production in the skin is triggered by UVB (short wavelengths). However, increased UVB exposure can lead to an increased risk of other sun-induced skin cancers, although these fortunately are often easier to treat and have a low mortality rate.

GETTING VITAMIN D FROM YOUR DIET.

You can derive a little vitamin D from your diet including fatty fish such as mackerel, cod liver oil, liver, eggs, milk and fortified margarine and breakfast cereals. However it is hard to derive sufficient vitamin D from dietary sources alone. It has been estimated that most adults are unlikely to derive more than five to 10 per cent of their vitamin D requirements from diet. For example, some food scientists have been able to boost vitamin D2 levels by 700% in button mushrooms by giving them a blast of UVB light! So get out there and absorb some sunshine.

That old favourite, cod-liver oil, is rich in vitamin D. One tablespoon provides 1,360 IU per serving compared to 566 IU in three ounces of swordfish and 41 IU in one egg yolk.

Researchers from the University of Surrey in the U.K. undertook an examination of the findings of 10 separate studies involving over 1,000 subjects to discover if vitamin D supplements are effective in raising vitamin D levels in humans.

Traditionally those foods fortified with the vitamin have used vitamin D2. However, vitamin D3 from eggs and oily fish has been found to be more effectively converted in the body for muscle and bone strength. This group is now examining whether food supplementation rather than stand-alone supplements could provide additional benefit whilst taking into consideration other variables including difference in gender, age, ethnicity and genetic make-up.

Recommendations for how much daily vitamin D is required depends on who you talk to! There is surprisingly little agreement between specialists as to what the optimal intake should be.

Currently the recommended intake suggests 200 IU daily for people up to age 50, 400 IU from ages 51 to 70, and 600 IU for those aged 71 and older. Other specialists suggest this is too low and we should obtain between 2,000 and 4,000 IU per day, ideally through a combination of sunlight exposure, diet and supplements. Certainly some individuals with obesity, osteoporosis, limited sunlight exposure or who have digestive or malabsorption problems would be advised to seek advice from their medical practitioner on any supplements and dosages.

RECOMMENDED DAILY INTAKE OF VITAMIN D

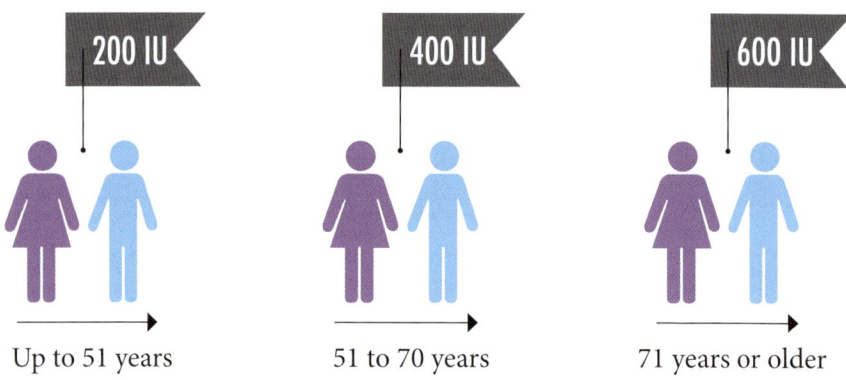

Up to 51 years   51 to 70 years   71 years or older

Vitamin D can be toxic in high levels and can cause risk of symptoms of anorexia, weight loss, passing too much urine (polyuria) and heart arrhythmias. Of greater concern, it can lead to elevated calcium levels, which may lead to increased calcification of blood vessels and tissue, causing potential damage to the heart, blood vessels and kidneys. Hence health professionals should always monitor supplementation.

Certainly vitamin D appears to play a major role in the health of the human body and brain.

There is a considerable amount of research being carried out investigating the role of vitamin D supplements for maintaining muscle strength and balance, particularly as we age. Vitamin D deficiency is now recognised as a cause of muscle weakness and muscle pain.

Other studies have found an association of low levels of vitamin D and the risk of certain cancers such as in the breast, colon, rectum, ovary, kidney, lung and uterus. Why this should be remains unclear, apart from the fact that vitamin D appears to help regulate cellular growth.

THE ROLE OF VITAMIN D AND COGNITION.

With a rapidly ageing population at risk of chronic medical disease and increasing physical frailty, it is essential to keep as well as possible as we age. With low levels of vitamin D now being reported globally, and its association with increased risk of impaired mobility, researchers are investigating levels of vitamin D in older adults.

In a British study by the Peninsula College of Medicine and Dentistry of over 2,000 people aged 65 and older, it was noted that as vitamin D levels went down, rates of cognitive impairment went up. Additional research on another 850 people had their cognitive functions measured using the Mini-Mental State Examination (MMSE), mental flexibility and mental speed. Subjects with severe deficiency compared to normal controls were 60% more likely to experience substantial general cognitive decline and 31% more likely to experience new problems with mental flexibility.

Other studies found similar findings in groups of older women, suggesting that vitamin D is linked to women's cognitive performance. One study from Angers in France and another from Minneapolis in the States found that in older women, higher dietary intake of vitamin D was associated with a lower risk of developing Alzheimer's, and, having lower levels of vitamin D was associated with a higher risk of global cognitive impairment and higher risk of global cognitive decline.

As you age, your ability to absorb vitamin D from sunlight diminishes, and if you are experiencing increasing physical frailty you may spend less time outside, which can compound the problem.

One idea that warrants further investigation is if the screening of older adults for vitamin D deficiency and treatment might be a way to minimise the future burden of cognitive impairment and dementia. The screening tests are relatively inexpensive and the treatment is also cheap.

If you believe you may be in a high-risk group for vitamin D deficiency, then why not talk to your doctor about arranging a blood test? Since low levels of vitamin D have no immediate associated symptoms, you may not know if your vitamin D levels are too low. Replacement using supplementation is always tailored to the level of insufficiency, and vitamin D concentrations should be monitored after three to four months.

Low levels of vitamin D are associated with an increased risk of cardiovascular disease, diabetes, depression, tooth decay, periodontal disease and osteoporosis, all of which are considered risk factors or have preceded the development of dementia.

Laboratory studies indicate that vitamin D plays a neuroprotective role in reducing inflammation. It is understood that inflammation is highly associated with the risk for both cardiovascular disease and Alzheimer's disease. In addition, vitamin D plays an important role in brain development and function.

Evidence is mounting that vitamin D may offer protection against auto-immune disorders through its anti-inflammatory effect and through strengthening the immune system. Type 1 diabetes, multiple sclerosis and rheumatoid arthritis fall into this category. In one study it was reported that women who supplemented their diet with 400 IU of vitamin D daily reduced their relative risk of multiple sclerosis by 40%.

VITAMIN D AND ALZHEIMER'S DISEASE.

Because vitamin D is associated with cognitive function, the question of whether low levels of vitamin D are associated with Alzheimer's disease led to a systemic review and meta-analysis of the data to date. The findings indicated that patients with Alzheimer's disease were shown to have low levels of vitamin D to a consistently significant degree, suggesting that the vitamin can in fact be viewed as a "neurosteroid" hormone and a potential biomarker of Alzheimer's.

The way Vitamin D3 may work appears to be by activating key genes and pathways that trigger the immune system to get rid of amyloid. Amyloid is one of the hallmarks of Alzheimer's disease and accumulates in what are called plaques in the brain. Turmeric is a compound currently being investigated because it has also been shown to assist in clearing beta amyloid from the brain. Using a combination of vitamin D with turmeric appears to boost the effect of the turmeric by enhancing the activity of specialised cells, called macrophages, which act as scavengers, actively engulfing amyloid.

A study from Kingston University in the U.K. compared the blood levels of vitamin D2 in patients diagnosed with Alzheimer's disease who were either receiving treatment with particular Alzheimer's medications or not. What they found was those people receiving treatment with drugs called anticholinesterase-inhibitors had higher levels of the vitamin. It is thought that the drugs switch back on the body's ability to absorb vitamin D somehow. As vitamin D2 is the storage form of the vitamin, the role of oily fish and egg yolks in the diet may prove useful here.

"...studies found that women with poor intake of vitamin D in middle age are adding to their potential risk of cognitive decline and Alzheimer's disease as they age."

Other studies found that women with poor intake of vitamin D in middle age are adding to their potential risk of cognitive decline and Alzheimer's disease as they age.

VITAMIN D AND PARKINSON'S DISEASE.

Parkinson's disease is a brain condition that affects around 2% of people over the age of 65, rising to 4-5% of 85-year-olds and older. It is the second most common form of neurodegenerative disease in Australia and remains one of the most poorly understood.

It is characterised by the loss of some highly specialised cells in an area of the brain called the substantia nigra. These cells are richly supplied with receptors for the neurotransmitter dopamine. Dopamine is widely used in the brain and has a number of roles including regulating mood, our ability to concentrate, and motivation (reward). In this area of the brain the dopamine is involved in controlling voluntary movement. Up to 80% of these specialised cells may have already been lost before the symptoms reveal themselves, which include:

- Tremors (often described in the hand as a pill-rolling tremor)
- Slowness of movement
- Difficulty in initiating movement
- Cognitive decline

Around 30% of people with Parkinson's disease will develop a form of dementia.

WHAT IS THE ROLE OF VITAMIN D IN PARKINSON'S DISEASE?

The role of vitamin D in Parkinson's disease is not fully understood. What is known from the research to date is that a higher level of vitamin D is associated with a lower risk of developing the condition. What can't be said yet is that there is any cause and effect relationship, just an association.

Finland is associated with low vitamin D levels in its population because of its latitude. The country conducted a study that revealed tested individuals with the highest levels of vitamin D were 67% less likely to develop Parkinson's disease, compared to those found to have the lowest levels. This study followed over 3,175 people aged 50 to 79 years over a 29-year period and so the results suggest that chronic vitamin D deficiency is a risk factor for Parkinson's disease. However it should also be noted that in this study, all the subjects had lower than the recommended levels of vitamin D, reflecting the widespread nature of the deficiency and the fact that deficiency is likely to be worse in a country that experiences relatively low levels of sunlight.

A different study published in 2010 in the prestigious journal JAMA (Journal of the American Medical Association) reported that individuals found to have a higher level of vitamin D were at a lower risk of developing Parkinson's disease.

Having a low level of vitamin D appears to be a risk factor for Parkinson's disease and the vitamin may have a neuro-protective effect via its antioxidant properties. Vitamin D is intimately associated with calcium and how our neurons conduct their messages.

The incidence of low levels of vitamin D is more prevalent in people diagnosed with Parkinson's disease compared even to individuals with Alzheimer's disease or the healthy elderly. A study from 2008 found that 55% of people diagnosed with Parkinson's disease had low levels of vitamin D compared to 41% of people with Alzheimer's and 36% of healthy adults.

The issue is that vitamin D insufficiency is recognised as a worldwide problem, even in sunny Australia. In a rapidly ageing population, it is also recognised that vitamin D production diminishes with age, at the very time when our brains would benefit from having sufficient amounts.

Researchers working with animal studies have suggested that the protective effect of vitamin D follows a U-shaped curve, implying there is a critical point at which the dose response will start to level off and even decline. This implies that there is an optimum dose for benefit. The trouble is the optimal dose remains unknown. So it cannot be currently recommended for people to take supplements of vitamin D unless their doctor has checked their blood levels, and treatment is considered appropriate.

VITAMIN D AND MULTIPLE SCLEROSIS.

Multiple sclerosis is a chronic condition of the brain and spinal cord, characterised by the patchy loss of the protective myelin sheath that surrounds both brain cell and spinal cord tracts. The presence of myelin enables electrical transmission along the nerve cells to travel at a much faster rate.

Currently there is no effective cure although some newer treatments are looking promising. The tragedy of multiple sclerosis is it tends to attack people in early middle age, just when they are at their peak of work and enjoying family life.

A study in 2011 noted that people who spent more time in the sun and had higher vitamin D levels had a lower risk of developing MS. Multiple sclerosis is more common in latitudes further away from the equator. However there is no link to suggest that low vitamin D in any way causes multiple sclerosis. In addition, those who have already been diagnosed with the condition do not benefit from vitamin D supplementation.

VITAMIN D AND DEPRESSION.

There are a number of studies examining the role of vitamin D and depression. However some of these have either been extremely small, e.g., three subjects, or used either very low doses of vitamin D in supplementation or very high doses. In addition, the findings have been quite inconsistent. So it has been difficult to get a sense of how valuable, if at all, vitamin D is for one's mood.

What determines our mood is subjective because there can be so many contributing factors. Many people say that having a little sunshine makes them feel better. Seasonal affective disorder or SAD is a recognised form of depression that people experience during times of the year when the days are shorter and there is less sunshine about. In the U.K., SAD occurs more in the winter months and then starts to disappear around spring time. Its aetiology is unclear but is thought to be associated with the effect of reduced light on a particular part of the brain called the hypothalamus and the amount of certain brain chemicals produced, including melatonin and serotonin.

University College of London in the U.K. published the results of a study that found low levels of vitamin D might be associated with an increased risk of depression in mid-life. The researchers commented that, "The high burden of mental and behavioural disorders and concurrent prevalence of vitamin D insufficiency <75nmlo/l worldwide highlights the potential importance of these findings."

In this study, data from 7,401 participants from the 1958 British birth cohort was analysed and revealed that at age 45, having a higher level of vitamin D was associated with lower levels of depression and panic. At age 50, a non-linear association between vitamin D and depression was revealed, with a lower risk for those people who had vitamin D levels between 50 and 85 nmol/l.

This builds on other research. For example, the third U.S. National Health and Nutrition Examination survey found that people with vitamin D deficiency were at an 85% increased risk of experiencing current episodes of depression compared to those with normal levels.

Bearing in mind that levels of vitamin D deficiency in the community are very high, as is the incidence of depression, it would appear prudent to check vitamin D levels and to monitor for symptoms of depression, as it is well recognised that in this high-risk group, depression can exacerbate a worse outcome of other medical conditions.

SMARTER THINKING: The prevalence of vitamin D insufficiency is extremely high worldwide. This has been associated with an increased risk of certain neurodegenerative conditions including Alzheimer's disease, Parkinson's disease and Multiple Sclerosis. While it is recognised that vitamin D is important for brain function and development, it also plays a role in maintaining mood. Getting your levels of vitamin D checked only requires a simple blood test, so why not chat to your health practitioner about getting it done?

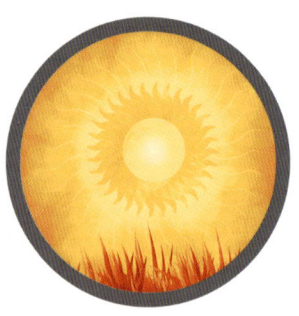

CHAPTER 5

ATTITUDE: MANAGE YOUR STRESS

WHAT IS STRESS?

For every person asked that question, there is likely a different answer. Stress is subject to interpretation because it depends on a person's unique experience and personality that defines what they find stressful. What some find nerve-racking may not cause another to blink an eye.

What a student finds stressful, for example, is dealing with the pressures of a lot of school work. For a business owner the stress may be from worry whether he can afford to pay the staff at the end of the week. For a farmer the stress may be from worrying about lack of rain and a poor harvest.

Whatever our interpretation of stress, it is how we deal with it that matters.

THE FIGHT-OR-FLIGHT RESPONSE

When we feel stressed there is a perceived threat to our well-being.

In the fight-or-flight response we have evolved so that when faced with a potential threat or danger, our body adapts physiologically to allow us to make a choice. We can stand and fight or we can run away as fast as possible.

If you are crossing a road and realise you are about to get mown down by a truck, it is probably better to choose to get out of the way real quick. In that split second, your heart rate and breathing rate increase, the blood flow to your limbs increases and your body pumps out hormones including adrenaline, noradrenaline and cortisol to maintain your body's state of readiness to escape harm.

If you have an important presentation to give, it's normal to experience some nervous energy in the same way. You may feel a bit anxious; have butterflies in the tummy or even nausea. But that heightened level of activity may serve you well in that particular

One of the really bad things about chronic, unmitigated stress is the effect it has on our brains.

situation to allow you to perform better. So in some cases, having a little bit of stress can be good for you.

The stress that isn't helpful is that horrid, gnawing, persistent worry that keeps you lying awake at night; unable to resolve the problem or situation you are trying to deal with.

The body is designed to allow us to flee or fight when danger presents itself. In Robert Sapolsky's book, Why Zebras Don't Get Ulcers, the point is that as a zebra on an African plain with a lion stalking the herd, you want to be able to run faster than the lion so you get out of the way and don't become his breakfast. Once that immediate danger is past, you can relax and go back to eating grass on the savannah. No long-term worry; just instant problem, instant solution.

Now if you were surrounded by a pack of hungry wolves and there was no sign of any of them giving up before they have ensured you are dinner, your body is under a continuing threat and the sustained elevated levels of stress hormones will start to damage your immune system and health (if the wolves didn't get you first)

One of the really bad things about chronic, unmitigated stress is the effect it has on our brains.

People who have first-hand experience of severe chronic stress will understand how difficult it is to focus on anything except the item that is worrying you. If you can't sleep or eat because of the stress you are experiencing, then your ability to focus and concentrate is reduced, you can't remember things and you can get pretty cranky, emotional and exhausted.

More than that, severe chronic stress through elevated cortisol levels has been shown to damage brain cells. It inhibits your brain's ability to form new connections between existing brain cells, or to produce new brain cells. It can cause the dendrites of existing brain cells to wither and disappear, so you lose existing connections.

In other words, this type of stress literally shrinks your brain. This is why it is so essential that in today's busy, demanding world you have effective stress management strategies in place when faced with a situation that could potentially cause a lot of stress, you are better positioned to handle it successfully.

HOW WE DEAL WITH STRESS

How we deal with stress is almost as varied as what causes us stress in the first place. There is no one solution to help everyone. Our different personalities and beliefs mean you can choose which method you feel most comfortable with and believe will be most helpful. You may even choose to use a combination of stress management methods. It's simply finding what works best for you.

RECOGNISING OUR "BRAIN DRAINERS"

There are a number of factors we may face on a daily basis which can be significant brain drainers. They hinder our ability to use our brains well or to function at the highest level.

These factors include:

- **Boredom and routine:** being stuck in a rut makes it more difficult to be engaged, to be creative or solution-focused.

- **Distractions:** we have multiple distractions of all kinds attacking us on a daily basis, taking away from the task we want to focus on. Managing these can be time-consuming and exhausting.

- **Multi-tasking:** the brain simply isn't designed to multi-task even though we like to kid ourselves that we can. If any one of those tasks requires our undivided attention, then all we are doing is using more brain energy and taking longer to complete tasks, while also making more errors.

- **Feeling overwhelmed:** just the sheer volume of work we can be expected to complete on a daily basis can lead to exhaustion, anxiety and stress-related illness.

- **Fatigue:** if we don't get enough sleep, our brains can't function properly.

- **Hunger:** it's hard to concentrate when your tummy is growling.

- **Negative attitude:** if we choose to support negative beliefs we are not allowing ourselves to expand our conscious thinking or be open to new ideas.

SMARTER THINKING: *Chronic stress causes damage to your brain. We are all different in our perceptions of and response to different stressors. By identifying what is causing your stress, you can take the first steps towards bringing it under control, allowing your brain to think better again. Choosing a method to manage stress is always a personal one and will depend on individual choice and circumstances.*

DEALING WITH DISTRACTIONS

Guilty as charged. It can often be a struggle to complete my daily tasks, as there is a constant stream of distractions vying for my attention. It's all too easy to get off-track and find that, at the end of the day, half the things you wanted to do aren't done simply because of all the interruptions and distractions that got in our way.

It's very easy to blame being busy and having to multi-task as excuses to cope with all of the demands put on us in our daily lives.

For example, I am easily distracted by the email in-box, unnecessary phone calls, children requiring pick-ups and even the demands of the dog. Whatever it is, I get very frustrated with my seemingly increasing inability to ignore everything and get the work done.

The fact is, as we get older our ability to cope with these distractions also diminishes. It's not so much that we can't focus; it's more that all the other stuff gets in the way. The result can be diminished short-term memory. And it's infuriating!

So, if this is a natural ageing process, what can we do to remedy the problem?

THE BRAIN HAS ITS OWN MECHANISM

Some very clever people at the Kavli Institute in Norway have discovered the brain actually has its own mechanism to allow us to filter out those distracting thoughts. Hooray! The key seems to be in the highly specialised area of the brain called the hippocampus, which deals with memory and learning.

 **OUR BRAIN CELLS CAN SELECT DIFFERENT BRAIN FREQUENCIES AND ARE CONSTANTLY CHANGING.**

The Kavli scientists used the analogy of a radio. When you really want to "tune in" to listen, you focus on what you want to hear and tune out the distractions of other noise. Our brains can do the same. The brain uses different frequencies of gamma waves to transmit diverse types of information, which can be past memories or current information like where you are right now. In the hippocampus, the brain cells can choose which frequency they want to focus on and, moreover, can switch to other frequencies very fast in just fractions of seconds.

This shows that our super plastic brains are probably even more malleable than we had first believed. We know that we can strengthen new neural pathways in our brains and allow others to diminish but this demonstrates an even greater flexibility is possible, whereby brain cells can select different brain frequencies and constantly change quickly.

CAN OLDER BRAINS ADAPT?

If we can learn to train our brains to ignore all those distractions more easily, then our concentration and short-term memory will benefit.

Attention training is a current trend gaining popularity in hopes of keeping one's mind sharp. Practising paying attention, even for a few minutes a day can bring long-lasting improvement.

There are a number of studies which have looked at cognitive brain training games but the suggestion is that even doing other brain activities such as Sudoku or crossword puzzles can help to reduce our susceptibility to distractions.

With brain games and cognitive training programs there is now an ever-increasing choice available. Some are even available on portable video game systems. Look for one that offers a graded set of activities that can be undertaken over a period of time that gradually get harder. Look for those that have a way you can test yourself as you progress, giving you a measurable idea of your improvement.

Participating in a regular or daily session of focused brain training or stimulation will pay off in better short-term memory and improved concentration, and I'm all for that!

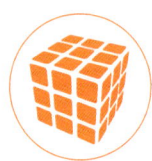

SMARTER THINKING: Brain games are not for everyone, so if you have a different form of brain activity you enjoy, do that! It's really important to choose one that appeals to you, is within your budget and that you will enjoy doing. There are lots to choose from, and the more varied the challenges, the more exercise for your brain.

WORK/LIFE BALANCE

In today's hurly-burly life, we are all suffering from a similar perception. The perception is that we are time-poor. Everything is a rush. We have more work, family commitments and demands than we have time for. It piles up on us like an avalanche: the kids need to be chauffeured to school and then to after school activities, the shopping has to be done, so do the household chores, there are bills to be paid, exercise to be fitted in somewhere and did anyone remember to feed the dog?

REMEMBER TO PRESS THE "PAUSE" BUTTON

Sometimes the days (and weeks and months), spin past us so fast that we lose sight of what is really important to us and forget to take the time to just STOP.

When you go away on holiday, do you take your mobile phone and your laptop to do work and be available? Hello! When did we all become so indispensable? The perceived need for constant contact 24/7 puts incredible pressure on us to do more, to work harder, for longer … for what?

When you are so busy, the brain is in constant overdrive. You are functioning on survival level. Your stress hormones are cranked up. You are trying to think, make decisions, and pursue your goals – without allowing time to relax sometimes and allow for creativity, reflection or deeper levels of thought.

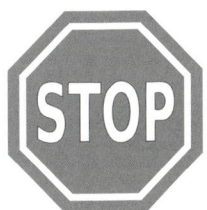

SOMETIMES THE DAYS (AND WEEKS AND MONTHS) SPIN PAST US SO FAST THAT WE CAN LOSE SIGHT OF WHAT IS REALLY IMPORTANT TO US AND FORGET TO TAKE THE TIME TO JUST STOP.

Hence, time to press the pause button.

I once saw a lady who was so stressed by her work overload she literally had become unable to think rationally about how to change her situation. She was on contract, earning good money, but totally exhausted from working over 18 months without any time off. Worse still, she was working full days then taking extra work home to finish off in the evening, sometimes continuing until 1 or 2 a.m. She always worked on the weekends too.

She recognised that her family and friends had stopped asking her out or inviting her to social functions, because she was always tied up with work or too exhausted to go. She was aware something needed to change, yet couldn't see how. She was scared that if she spoke to her employer he would simply replace her with someone else willing to do the work. Her fear and her exhausted brain stopped her from seeking alternative solutions to her situation.

And she is not alone. Many small business owners, executives, and employees are working under enormous levels of stress.

The bad news is that this is really bad for our brains. Stress is toxic to brain cells.

Have you ever felt the sort of worry that keeps you awake at night, an intense stress that either prevents you from eating anything or drives you to overeat? If so, you will likely already know how hard it is to see the bigger picture when weighed down by problems and worries.

Problems at home can be particularly difficult to put aside and sometimes additional errors and mistakes are made because we are unable to pay attention or focus. In business, this ultimately costs time or money or perhaps even your job if you fail to manage your stress.

Too often, all our focus is on working in the business without time being factored in to work on the business. This includes taking time just to stop and think about priorities, goals, values and beliefs. It might mean actually closing down your shop for a few days to give yourself breathing space and provide an opportunity to come back to work with a fresh approach.

What do you want to achieve with your work or business? What do you yearn for on behalf of your partner, your kids? Is it more money, more time, more balance?

As a general practitioner I used to see many people struggling everyday with simply too much on their plate. Their high stress levels were a huge cost to their mental and physical health.

I repeat, stress is toxic to brain cells. It stops your brain cells from forming new connections so you are unable to learn or remember new information. Your memory retrieval drops off, your concentration span is reduced, and you are off track. You have an increased risk of mental illness, anxiety, depression, panic attacks and burnout. Physically you are then at increased risk of developing heart disease, hypertension and cancer.

Too often, all our focus is on working in our business or in our lives, without allowing time to work on the business or on our lives. This includes taking time to stop and think about our priorities, goals, values and beliefs.

So, remember to hit the pause button.

Remind yourself:

- it's okay to sometimes say "No" or "Stop"

- It's okay to decide not to work the extra overtime

- It's okay to take a real holiday minus the phone, computer and other devices that chain us to our work

 **SMARTER THINKING:** *It can be liberating to come back from leave and discover the earth is still turning, the office didn't self-combust and your customers haven't all abandoned you. Maybe there are some steps you can take to give yourself a little valuable time off.*

SWEET DREAMS

You may have experienced the effect of enjoying a really late night and then finding the next day how hard it is not only to stay awake but also to pay attention and focus.

As you get older, your capacity to deal with sleep deprivation seems to diminish as well. Without proper sleep, your susceptibility to stress increases. A proper night's sleep is vital to our health and a healthy attitude!

SLEEP IS ESSENTIAL FOR GOOD BRAIN HEALTH

We all need sleep, but many of us are chronically sleep-deprived. This can reduce mental performance on a daily basis, decreasing one's ability to cope with stress, lowering resistance to infection because your immune system is impaired, and aggravating the risk of developing chronic disease.

The amount of sleep we get each night varies with individuals and age. There is no right amount. The average varies between six and ten hours. Some people can manage on less than others. You may have heard the anecdotes of people such as Margaret Thatcher who manage to get by on as little as four hours of sleep per night. Others may need a full eight hours in order to have some chance of functioning normally. Typically, infants and growing children need the greatest amount.

As we age, we get by on less sleep, although our sleep patterns may also be disrupted by medication or pain (e.g., arthritis). If we have depression, have had a stroke or have cognitive impairment, our sleep may also be disordered.

CAN WE CATCH UP ON SLEEP?

Will a long sleep-in on the weekend help if we've been sleep-deprived during the week? The short answer is no.

This is a common pattern for many people where work and other commitments can cause us to go to bed later than planned, so we are tired the next morning. Unfortunately, sleeping in on the weekend is not usually sufficient to pay back our sleep debt, so we become more chronically sleep-deprived.

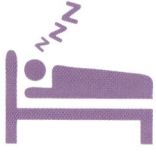 AS YOU GET OLDER, YOUR CAPACITY TO DEAL WITH SLEEP DEPRIVATION SEEMS TO DIMINISH AS WELL. WITHOUT PROPER SLEEP, YOUR SUSCEPTIBILITY TO STRESS INCREASES. A PROPER NIGHT'S SLEEP IS VITAL TO OUR HEALTH AND A HEALTHY ATTITUDE!

Studies have shown that the effects of chronic sleep deprivation produce the same effects on performance as drinking alcohol. When you are tired your reaction times start to slow down. A normal reaction time of around quarter of a second can double in length when you are really tired. It is also possible in fatigue to experience micro-sleep, where we literally zone out for a couple of seconds. If this was to occur while driving, it could produce disastrous consequences.

Have you ever found yourself driving without thought due to lack of sleep or exhaustion to suddenly find yourself barely avoiding a dangerous situation, such as running a red light at an intersection, because you had fallen asleep for just a moment? Or have you arrived at your destination without any memory of actually driving there? It can be frightening to see the errors of our judgement first-hand, purely because one's foggy, sleep-deprived brain was not its usual vigilant self.

We spend roughly one third of our lives asleep and 80% of that is true deep sleep, which is associated with slow brain waves. Think about it: if the average person lives for 80 years, that's nearly 26 years of our lives spent asleep!

WHY DO WE NEED TO SLEEP?

Perhaps there is no hard evidence, but there are a number of theories as to why the human body and brain need to sleep.

- Sleep allows time for the brain to rest, for neurons to repair and regenerate, to get rid of waste and be able to function better when we wake.

- This down time helps the brain consolidate and retain information. The brain replays the day's events and helps form long-term memories.

- Deep sleep seems to give the brain time to strengthen existing synaptic connections and to weaken others, allowing the brain to let go of information no longer needed.

It is proven that sleep deprivation is associated with a negative effect on our thinking and health. Many people suffer some form of disrupted sleep patterns or insomnia.

In one study of middle-aged men with sleep disturbances, it was found that they had higher levels of cortisol and corticotropic hormone (CRH). These hormones are associated with the fight-or-flight response. In other words, their brains were in a heightened level of arousal resulting in a poorer quality of sleep.

If you are a "brooder" or a worrier or someone who tends to react emotionally to problems, you may be the one tossing and turning at night, unable to sleep as your brain keeps replaying the same problem loop in your head.

If you can keep the emotions at bay it is possible to sleep on a problem. With sufficient deep sleep you are better able to problem solve and wake with a solution. Eureka!

Sleep deprivation can lead to:

- Cognitive impairment, decline in memory and judgement, poor attention
- Increased risk of depression
- Higher risk of diabetes and heart disease
- Reduced immune function
- Increased risk of obesity

WHAT HAPPENS IN THE BRAIN WHEN WE SLEEP?

The sleep cycle can be broken down into five separate stages. We move from stage one, where you we are just falling asleep, to stage two, where we spend 60% of the sleep cycle. We then slip into stages three and four of deep sleep, where the brain shows slow waves and the final stage is called Rapid Eye Movement (REM) sleep, which lasts for 20 to 25% of each sleep cycle. REM sleep is when we tend to do most of our dreaming.

 **EACH SLEEP CYCLE LASTS AROUND 90 MINUTES AND SO, ON A TYPICAL NIGHT, WE WILL GO THROUGH FIVE OR SIX ENTIRE CYCLES.**

Each sleep cycle lasts around 90 minutes and so, on a typical night, we will go through five or six entire cycles. It seems that the different stages of sleep are all important for different aspects of one's memory.

At the end of one sleep cycle and as you go into a lighter sleep you may either wake up or enter another cycle all over again. Typically, you spend more time in the slow wave sleep in the earlier part of the night and longer periods in the REM cycle towards early morning. This slow wave type of sleep is associated with brain learning, the "how-to" process associated with learning a musical instrument or decision-making.

SLEEP PROBLEMS

If you are suffering through a temporary situation (like having a newborn baby in the house) that will pass, sometimes you can get through it by taking advantage of naps and early bedtimes.

If, however, the problem is really entrenched, it's time to seek help. Medication with sleeping tablets really only offers a short-term benefit and may compound the problem if overused. Longer-term management requires looking into all factors that may hinder getting a good night's sleep. We call this "sleep hygiene."

GOOD SLEEP HABITS INCLUDE:

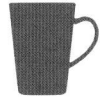

1. Reducing caffeine. Everyone knows drinking coffee late at night may keep you awake. But perhaps we are consuming too much caffeine over the day as well. That cup of coffee at lunchtime could be enough to disturb your sleep that night. The half-life of caffeine is six hours, so try not to have caffeine within eight hours of going to sleep if you are sensitive to its effect.

Caffeine is found in tea (black and green), chocolate and cola drinks. The popular "energy drinks" with guarana such as Red Bull and Mother have very high caffeine levels.

So the first thing to do is to reduce or, ideally, eliminate the amount of caffeine you drink. Include more non-caffeine beverages such as herbal brews of camomile, fennel and anise, and drink plenty of water.

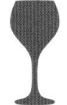

2. Avoid alcohol. Alcohol, which appears to relax us and does get us off to sleep, is unfortunately associated with a poorer quality of sleep so you are more likely to wake up in the night.

3. Relax. Going to bed in a relaxed mood will help you get off to sleep. Having a warm bath and a drink of hot milk (the tryptophan in the warm milk is a natural sleep inducer) can settle your mind and put you in a calm state for sleeping.

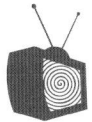

4. Turn off the TV. Take it out of the bedroom, preferably. You want to avoid overstimulating the brain, so switch it off.

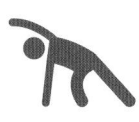

5. Exercise. Twenty to thirty minutes of exercise each day (as a minimum) helps us to sleep better at night, but don't do it too late in the evening, otherwise it will have the opposite effect. If you exercise in the evening, make sure you're finished at least three hours before you want to go to sleep.

6. **Have a regular bedtime**. Going to bed and getting up at the same time every day encourages good sleep patterns. So work out a routine that suits you and stick to it.

7. **Can't sleep? Get up.** If you really can't sleep it's better to physically get up, have a cup of warm milk or read a book until you feel naturally sleepy again and then go back to bed.

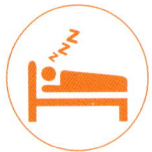

SMARTER THINKING: *Getting enough uninterrupted sleep is crucial for good brain health. Far from being at rest at night, when you sleep your brain is encoding memory and maintaining and repairing brain cells ready to fire up for the next day.*

HAVE A LAUGH

As Woody Allen said:
"I am grateful for laughter except when the milk comes out of my nose."

When did you last have a good laugh? You know, one of those really good, deep belly laughs where we temporarily become engulfed in an uncontrollable fit of the giggles. The one where our bodies shake helplessly in spasms, with tears pouring down our faces. Where we become unable to think or do anything until the moment is gone and our outpouring of guffaws, snorts or hoots has passed.

And how do we feel afterwards? Relaxed? Exhausted? Likely, we feel happy and have a more positive outlook on life.

LAUGHTER LOWERS STRESS

After a release of laughter, our problems and worries don't seem so big or scary anymore. Our resilience to life's challenges improves.

And that's why laughter is so good for our brains. We think better, have increased memory capacity, improved focus and attentiveness and are more positive when we include laughter in our lives.

When we laugh, a variety of different areas in the brain light up in activity. Our logical left-brain analyses the words we hear or the situation we're in. This activates our frontal lobes looking to organise and plan. The right hemisphere "gets the big picture" and then our sensory and motor areas become involved as well. Many areas of the brain are involved in quite distinct neural pathways when we laugh.

Laughter lowers levels of cortisol and adrenaline, the so-called stress hormones, and increases endorphin levels. Less cortisol helps us feel happy and less prone to anxiety or depression. It helps us keep a better perspective on things going on in our lives. Was that bad event really so terrible?

When you laugh, your blood pressure changes. First it increases and then drops as you engage in deeper breathing and this helps to send more oxygenated blood to your brain.

Laughter can also be an expression of relief. Have you ever noticed that when you have had to deal with a serious or emotionally draining situation that the tension can be relieved by having a laugh afterwards?

LAUGHTER CREATES CONNECTION

At school or in areas where we have to absorb and learn new information, have you noticed it is those teachers who engage their students with fun and excitement in their lessons who make the whole learning experience much more memorable?

When studying or working hard, taking time out with friends to share a laugh or a joke will help us to engage better with learning and remembering too. We can focus and concentrate better – essential prerequisites for memory.

Children laugh so much more than we do as adults. Kids laugh up to 300 times a day! Adults are lucky if we manage 17 laughs a day.

Where did all that fun go?

What is one of the first social cues we look for in our newborn babies?

That's right, the first smile. That first toothless grin is such a magic moment, bonding infant with parent. When we hear babies and children laughing, we are more likely to laugh too.

If you are feeling down or in need of cheering up, have you ever decided to find a comedy show on the TV or gone to watch a funny film? Why do we choose to do this? It's because we know from experience that if we do, it provides us with a temporary escape from all the other stuff in our lives that may be overwhelming us, making us sad, depressed or anxious. Using comedy to lighten our moods makes us feel better overall.

Remember, laughter is infectious. Catch one person laughing and the mood in the whole room will lift and others will join in as well. It bonds people sharing the experience and improves the group's ability to communicate better. Even if we don't share the same language, a shared laugh crosses all barriers.

HOW CAN YOU BRING MORE JOY INTO YOUR LIFE?

First up, choose to do so. Look for opportunities to lighten up, maybe not take yourself so seriously and let go. Relax!

Practise smiling.

- Make a conscious effort to smile and acknowledge people. (Even if, and especially if, you are not in the mood for it!)

- Smile at the checkout person in the supermarket. (And they are sometimes in serious need of a smile!)

- Smile at random strangers. So what if they think you are nuts? They will think you are a happy person and they may even smile back. And every smile you receive back will lift your mood.

When taking the dog out for an early morning walk, or going to the gym or doing exercise in the park, smile at everyone you meet. By the time you get to work you will have already exchanged smiles with half a dozen or more people. You are likely to be in a much better frame of mind to start your day.

Smiles defuse tension and anxiety. They provide support and show someone you care.

It takes more muscles to smile, so give your face a workout and smile often!

Spend time with others who make you smile and who enjoy humour in their own lives. Sharing a joke with friends builds connections and allows us to express our true feelings more.

There are even laughter classes now. The medical and social benefits of laughter have been recognised as being so beneficial that trained laughologists (no, really!) run classes with the purpose of reducing stress, raising energy levels, making your outlook more positive and strengthening your immune system. Laughter triggers the brain to release endorphins, the feel-good chemicals that help us to achieve a sense of well-being. Our levels of dopamine and serotonin increase and our levels of cortisol decrease.

The study of laughter is called gelatology (sounds to me like ice cream) and I'd like two scoops of that, please.

Dr. "Patch" Adams in the U.S. is well known for his use of humour and laughter as a way of helping people heal when they have been sick. Humour has been found to reduce the amount of pain experienced by patients when recovering. Which would you rather have? A couple of painkillers, or a shot of humour?

Studies have shown that watching a comedy program rather than a drama allows blood vessel walls to relax, increasing blood flow and oxygen flow to our brains and reducing blood pressure.

And don't forget, we tend to be more attracted to people we perceive as having a good sense of humour. So, what's a simple way to be perceived as an attractive person with a great personality? You got it. Let go, and have a good laugh.

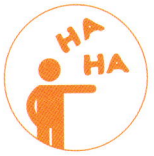

SMARTER THINKING: *Laughter is a brilliant stress buster and makes us more attractive to other people. If having a laugh helps us to enjoy life more, then we could all benefit from seeking to add more fun and joy into everything we do every day.*

BE SOCIAL

Being lonely is not good for us. People on the whole are social beings and we thrive on contact and interaction with others.

How vivid is that image of an older person living alone, with little or no social contact? Apart from the disadvantage of being socially isolated, that person is also significantly at risk of increased physical and mental ill health and is likely to age faster and die earlier.

WHY IS SOCIALISING IMPORTANT FOR BRAIN HEALTH AND BETTER MEMORY SKILLS?

The incidence of mental illness, including depression, is more common in those living alone.

Studies have demonstrated that people on their own are less likely to maintain good cognitive function and have a higher risk of developing dementia.

Less external stimulation means less engagement with what is happening in the rest of the world, less likelihood of expanding or learning new mental skills, or of remaining interested and curious about the life around them.

Having to use your brain in a social sense means using your memory to remember, controlling your emotions (both positively and negatively) and being attentive and focused.

Neuroscience has taught us that in order to remain brain fit we need to actively flex all of our mental muscle. Much advice is centred on engaging in new and varied intellectual activities. However, a number of studies have found that remaining socially engaged is just as important in maintaining our cognitive health.

In 2007, Professor Oscar Ybarra and his colleagues released a paper that looked to prove a correlation between social engagement and better brain function. His study included 3,600 people between the ages of 24 and 65. He analysed data on how often people talked on the phone to friends, how often they got together socially with family or friends and how many people they felt close enough with to discuss private matters or concerns. He found that across all age groups, the more socially engaged the participants were, the better their working (short term) memories. They also had a lower risk of cognitive impairment.

In a different study of 2,000 Middle-Eastern older adults, he again showed a strong correlation between social engagement and being able to make day-to-day decisions. Ybarra believes the human mind has evolved to deal with social problems.

In a third study, with a group of 18- to 21-year-olds, he demonstrated that social interaction produced better cognitive performance. In this study there were three groups. The first group was engaged in a discussion for 10 minutes. The second group performed brain-training activities (crossword puzzles/Sudoku) for 10 minutes. The third group sat and watched a 10-minute Seinfeld clip. The groups were then tested on speed of processing information and working memory.

The results showed that even after only a 10-minute exercise, the group involved in the discussion did far better in working memory tests than those who had watched the video clip. The brain-training group was a close second to the discussion group.

So, talking and social interaction with your fellow human beings appears very important in being able to maintain good cognitive function, even more than doing the brain-training programs. Altho gh they are, of course, also recognised for contributing in a big way to our improvement of cognitive function.

It looks as if we have another good reason to turn off the TV.

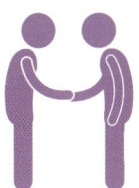 TALKING AND SOCIAL INTERACTION WITH YOUR FELLOW HUMAN BEINGS APPEARS VERY IMPORTANT IN BEING ABLE TO MAINTAIN GOOD COGNITIVE FUNCTION, EVEN MORE THAN DOING THE BRAIN-TRAINING PROGRAMS.

REDUCED SOCIAL CONTACT IS A GROWING CONCERN

The need for human beings to remain connected to each other is important for a number of reasons. The above study suggests that having better social skills means we are more likely to enjoy a better cognitive outcome. This means that if our kids are taught good social skills from an early age then they are likely to perform better academically.

In the workplace, these skills can be developed in others by encouraging employee interactivity and socialising as a way to help them work better and more productively.

However, our changing lifestyle means many more of us now choose to live alone. The family unit is being replaced by an increasing number of single person units.

There has also been a big increase in the number of people choosing to work from home as solopreneurs, as virtual assistants or in online businesses, without any personal contact with other staff or related personnel.

Additionally there are a large number of baby boomers reaching retirement age who, either through choice, divorce or the death of their partners are likely to end up living alone.

If we want our brains to keep working and reduce the risk of losing our memory skills, our physical and our overall mental health, it is crucial we all maintain or increase our social networks.

Younger people living alone may be more likely to continue to engage with other younger people, but we need to look out for the shy, the geeky or the socially introverted personalities.

For people living and working from home, it takes some effort to ensure we get out and interact with others, to have some face-to-face meetings, to socialise with friends, to go to restaurants and cafés – contact beyond just having a chat with the cashier in the check-out queue of the supermarket.

For the elderly, physical infirmity can be a major issue, making it harder to get out and remain connected.

As a general practitioner I looked after a number of elderwly people who were sick or infirm and living alone. Quite often it would only be the Silver Chain nurse, the Meals on Wheels delivery person or myself paying a visit that provided them with any social contact with the outside world.

Maintaining inter-generational contact is also important. Elderly people have been shown to maintain better cognition and mood if they have contact with younger people.

Enjoying rich and meaningful relationships with fellow human beings remains an essential part of maintaining good cognitive performance. Apart from keeping us from depression, we are better able to think more clearly and remember things better.

GET OUT OF THE HOUSE MORE OFTEN

It makes sense that being engaged in activities with others leads to us feeling healthier and less prone to depression. Going out to meet friends, enjoying restaurant meals, going to the cinema, the theatre or a museum is more likely to give people a sense of well-being and make them more resistant to depression. This has been verified by a Norwegian study of over 48,000 people and it was true regardless of socio-economic background, general health, or smoking and alcohol use.

Regardless of our individual social situations, there are a number of things we can consider to remain socially connected, such as:

- Joining community groups
- Maintaining regular social contact with friends
- Going out to social functions, clubs
- Travelling and going on holiday

- Enrolling for courses at the local Tafe college or university
- Being a volunteer for a charity or other community group
- Having a dog that requires a walk outside

Even the telephone can provide a means of at least speaking to another person, as can social media channels like Facebook, Twitter and Skype.

One of my former clients was a widow with no children. Yet she had a wide circle of friends who visited regularly; she entertained most weeks, held regular lunch and supper parties and used the phone to connect with friends who lived further away. She also took a keen interest in staying up-to-date with what was going on in the world. She was mentally sharp as a tack and even took computer lessons to learn how to send email. Not bad for a 96-year-old.

SMARTER THINKING: *Being socially active has a major effect on your health and well-being. Throughout your lifetime there is nothing that can replace the invaluable act of simply being with and interacting with another person every day to provide great mental exercise.*

MEDITATION

Over the centuries, meditation has been used to reduce stress, improve focus, attention and memory.

A few years ago, I enrolled in a six-week meditation course. And I have to say it was hugely beneficial. Having to mentally and physically stop for that one brief hour each week was very calming and it did help me cope.

I can't say it was easy, either. Being a person always on the go, never allowing myself the luxury to step back and stop the endless mind-chatter was quite a challenge and it took a while to get the hang of it. But then I would start to look forward to that time, and little by little I did learn how to focus on the breath, to be more present and just take in the sounds around me without allowing my thoughts to rudely intrude and distract. I could actually just acknowledge them and let them float off somewhere else.

Whilst there is a lot of awareness of the beneficial physiological changes associated with meditation, it has only been over the last few years that scientific studies have been able to show more of what is going on in the brain when we meditate, and the promise of what further research may bring for future brain health benefits.

The brain itself actually undergoes physical change in response to meditation.

A study by Sara Lazar, research scientist from the Massachusetts Hospital in Boston, showed that regular meditation causes thickening of the cerebral cortex in those areas of the brain associated with decision-making, attention and memory.

The question arising from her study is: would regular meditation slow the natural thinning of the cortex that occurs with age?

The cortex is associated with higher brain function. So, can meditation increase attention span, sharpen focus and improve memory?

The proponents of meditation say it can.

In 2007, a study by Amishi Jha and Michael Baine at Penn's Stress Management Program at the University of Pennsylvania looked at how meditation affected the three separate components of paying attention, i.e.:

- The ability to prioritise and manage tasks and goals

- The ability to voluntarily focus on specific information

- The ability to stay alert to the environment

They had two test groups. The first group was new to meditation and undertook an eight-week course, which included 30 minutes of daily meditation. The second group was experienced in meditation and went on a full time, one-month retreat.

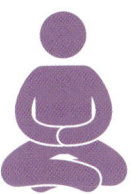

THE BRAIN ACTUALLY UNDERGOES PHYSICAL CHANGE IN RESPONSE TO MEDITATION.

Both groups underwent computer-based tests on response speeds and accuracy, and both groups showed improved performance in attention and ability to focus. The experienced group did better overall but the new group demonstrated significant improvement over the course of just a few weeks.

The implications here suggested it would be worthwhile teaching employees to meditate, because even 30 minutes a day can produce improved attention and focus.

Attention is the key to learning. So it would appear that meditation allows you to improve your attention and hence, your learning capacity.

The Deutsche Bank, Google, and Hughes Aircraft now offer meditation classes for their workers because of the perceived benefits to their employees, including:

- Increased productivity
- Reduced stress-related illness
- Reduced absenteeism
- Reduced number of errors or mistakes
- Improved recall and memory due to a relaxed and clear mind

Mental activity in meditation is both wakeful and relaxed. Professor Jim Lagopoulos from Sydney University used electroencephalogram (EEG) testing to look at the differences in the brain when mentally active, resting, asleep or meditating, as the brain has some form of electrical activity in all of these states.

He found that those engaged in non-reactive meditation produced more marked changes in electrical brain wave activity associated with wakeful relaxed attention, compared to those who were just resting without any specific mental technique.

IS MEDITATION A GOOD TOOL TO PREVENT MEMORY LOSS?

The results of a small pilot study that looked into the use of meditation to prevent memory loss were published in March, 2010 by Dr. Dharma Singh Khalsa, and Andrew Newberg (an associate professor of radiology at the Pennsylvania University School of Medicine).

They had 15 subjects with known memory problems, aged between 52 to 77 years. They undertook eight weeks of Kirtan Kriya mediation for 12 minutes a day and had all undergone cognitive testing and brain imaging at the beginning and end of the eight-week period.

The meditation method used was very simple. The subjects had to repeat four sounds: *sa, ta, na,* and *ma,* while touching their thumbs sequentially to their index, middle, ring and little fingers.

They had to perform this out loud for two minutes, at a whisper for two minutes, in silence for four minutes, then a whisper for two minutes and finally out loud again for two minutes.

Next, they were all given a meditation CD to play at home.

A control group of seven people with memory loss were asked just to listen to two Mozart violin concertos for 12 minutes a day.

Of the 15 in the meditation group:

- 7 had mild age-associated memory impairment
- 5 had mild cognitive impairment
- 3 had moderate impairment with Alzheimer's disease.

Of the five in the control group:

- 2 had mild cognitive impairment
- 3 had age-related memory impairment.

When subjects were scanned, the results found that those in the meditating group showed increased blood flow to frontal and parietal lobes (areas associated with memory retrieval). In cognitive testing, they all had improved performance in general memory and attention.

Those in the control group who had listened to music showed some increased blood flow in different areas of the brain but of less significance, and they showed no improvement in cognition.

The suggestion from the study is that meditation may be useful to those with mild memory impairment to slow down or inhibit progression of memory loss by "strengthening" the brain.

Whilst interesting, it has to be noted that this was an extremely small study, but certainly warrants further investigation with larger studies to see if this finding can be replicated.

Other researchers have also looked at the question of whether meditation can assist focus and thereby allow better memory.

Dr. Gary W. Small, director of the Memory and Ageing Research Centre, University of California has found that exposing older people to technology such as the internet changed their brain activity in just one week. He found that the older subjects showed an increase in frontal lobe activity and also in other areas of the brain where short term memory and decision-making are important.

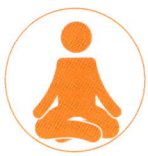

SMARTER THINKING: *Meditation appears to be a useful tool not only for the workplace but also to perhaps assist us in maintaining our cognition as we get older. It may not be too long before meditation is offered more widely as a strategy to keep us brain fit.*

MINDFULNESS TRAINING

There are a number of occupations that often expose workers to high levels of extreme stress. Think about the Olympic athletes who have spent months and years preparing for those few special minutes that could lead to the ultimate dream of winning an Olympic medal.

What about the police, ambulance officers and paramedics who are sent out to deal with major road traffic accidents, or the aid and health workers who provide help in natural disasters such as the earthquake in Haiti? They face stressful situations daily. Then of course, there are the soldiers deployed to war zones, living and working in highly dangerous areas, and each day facing the potential risks to their own lives.

It takes a certain type of person who is willing to embrace and take on this type of work, and it is well recognised they are doing so with great sacrifice and personal risk to their own physical or mental well-being.

We know that stress damages brain cells. There have been reports of high levels of post-traumatic stress disorder and mental illness in soldiers returning from war. Continued exposure to high levels of stress triggers sustained cortisol release, which can lead to a lessened ability to be able to think quickly and effectively and make well-thought-out decisions.

One study looked at how mental fitness can be improved by using mindfulness training in a group of soldiers prior to their deployment to Iraq.

Soldiers have to be physically fit. They undergo rigorous training to ensure they are at their peak of physical fitness. This study looked at whether increasing their mind fitness would produce soldiers better equipped to deal emotionally and mentally with the demands of modern warfare.

WHAT IS MINDFULNESS TRAINING?

Mindfulness is the ability to be aware and attentive of the present moment without any emotional reaction.

If you can practice mindfulness you may be able to avoid panic in a dangerous or difficult situation. You can evaluate and respond in a rational, logical way to produce the best outcome. This ability is immensely valuable to anyone, not just those exposed to extreme stress.

In the study, the group of soldiers who engaged in the mindfulness training over an eight-week period developed an increased capacity of their working memory, and reduced negative mood.

This would suggest that mindfulness training may be of significant value to all involved in high stress occupations. Those who work in other high pressure environments, in the corporate sector for example, would also benefit from such training.

Even beyond the high stress environment, the value of an increasing awareness of the benefits of mindfulness training would seem logical and is a potential means of improving psychological resilience for the working population at large.

WHAT ARE THE SKILLS OF MINDFULNESS TRAINING?

By being aware of the current moment, you can be much more focused and able to concentrate on the job at hand. People talk about being "in the zone" whereby they enjoy that higher level of focus and concentration, they can anticipate outcomes better, and their work just seems to flow with less effort.

BY BEING AWARE OF THE CURRENT MOMENT, YOU CAN BE MUCH MORE FOCUSED AND ABLE TO CONCENTRATE ON THE JOB AT HAND.

It helps with managing and avoiding distractions. Remaining focused on the now doesn't allow past experience to interfere. It also allows the emotional baggage to be kept under control. One can learn to notice the emotion but not allow it to interfere with the decision-making process. With practice it becomes easier to recognise when our thoughts are being governed by our emotions and to give them space rather than reacting immediately to the emotional trigger, in much the same way that we count to ten or walk away when angry. By keeping stress out of the picture, the person practising mindfulness may feel more relaxed and in a more positive mood.

SEEK HELP

Unresolved stress damages your brain and is toxic to brain cells. It can also lead to more serious mental health issues of anxiety and depression. If you think you may be suffering from this, please seek help. There are a number of professional and organizational sources you can contact, as well as reaching out to your personal circle of friends and family. If you are concerned about someone else who may be suffering from anxiety and depression, first just ask if they are okay. Talk to them and if it appears they are in trouble, suggest they seek help.

SMARTER THINKING: Mindfulness training is a powerful way to learn how to approach difficult or challenging situations in such a way that, by removing any attached emotion, possible solutions become much more obvious more quickly.

MANAGING ANXIETY

Anxiety is that uncomfortable feeling we get sometimes when we are nervous. We may feel jittery, sweaty, and breathless, and feel our hearts pound in our chests. We are in high alert and may find it hard to sit still. It puts us in the realm of "what if": what if something goes wrong, what if I make a mistake, what if I get fired, what if the doctor gives me bad news, what if I don't pass the exam or any number of upsetting scenarios.

Most of us can usually cope with brief doses of anxiety. Performance anxiety is common before walking onto a stage to sing or speak. Waiting for the start gun for a race creates a sense of anxiety that is quickly resolved by getting on with the race. It is often the anticipation that is associated with the anxiety.

Sometimes however, that sense of anxiety doesn't drop away but stays with us.

Having increased levels of anxiety over a period of time can lead to weight loss and a general feeling of inability to cope, not just with whatever is making us feel anxious (assuming we can identify it), but life in general.

If left unchecked, high levels of anxiety impair your ability not only to think clearly, but to think rationally. Panic disorder is a serious condition, which can lead to a person becoming disabled, unable to cope with "normal" day-to-day activities or work.

How we cope with anxiety depends on our individual resilience and life skills. Listening to relaxation tapes, walking and meditating are all ways to help. Sometimes just talking to a close friend, family member, or counsellor will make a difference and help us work out how we can best manage our anxiety levels.

Anxiety is very common. Many of us may not readily admit to having difficulties with anxiety and depression, but you are not alone. Over 40 million Americans are estimated to suffer from anxiety every year. There's a fine balance between what we can normally cope with on a day-to-day basis to being tipped over the edge. It can be difficult sometimes to identify what causes us to go from keeping on top of life's challenges to mental and physical breakdown.

Between 10% and 15% of the population are likely to experience depression at some point in their lives.

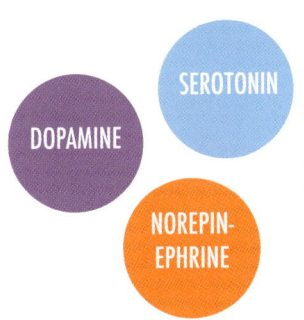

THREE MAIN BRAIN CHEMICALS

HELP MAINTAIN A NORMAL MOOD

COPING WITH DEPRESSION

Winston Churchill described his depression as his "black dog." Between 10% to 15% of the population are likely to experience depression at some point in their lives. It can affect people in all walks of life.

Having a mental illness such as depression has less social stigma than it used to, yet many people still find it hard to admit that they've had a depressive illness. Often this is because of their perceived negative reaction from friends or colleagues.

The diagnosis and management of depression has improved greatly and most people receive effective treatment that allows them to make a full recovery.

WHAT IS DEPRESSION?

Depressed people experience a mixture of symptoms and feelings including sadness, apathy and lack of motivation. They may have lost interest in things they would normally enjoy. They may withdraw from friends and family.

Sleep can be disturbed, too. Sufferers of depression may have difficulty getting to sleep or being unable to get up in the morning. Libido can be reduced or lost. Appetite may be lost or gained, leading to changes in body weight.

Depression was first considered to be a result of unhappy life events or stress. However the causes are now thought to be somewhat more complex and may also be a result of the interplay between genetic and environmental factors. Other factors include gender, illness, personality, stress and age.

There are three main brain chemicals or neurotransmitters that help us to maintain a normal mood. These are serotonin, dopamine and norepinephrine.

In depression, the levels of neurotransmitters are suppressed.

THE ROLE OF SEROTONIN

The serotonin in our brains plays an important role in determining how we think, behave and react emotionally.

It is a neurotransmitter passing across the synapses between nerve cell endings. Having a lower-than-normal level of serotonin has been associated with the development of depression, hence many of today's antidepressant medications are designed to help restore serotonin levels to normal.

A particular transporter protein for serotonin is responsible for the re-uptake of serotonin in the synapse. A gene that makes this transporter protein has been identified and there is one particular form of this gene that, if inherited, means the person has four times the risk of developing stress-related depression.

But it is more complex than just being at increased risk of inheriting one gene. Another gene, the brain-derived neurotrophic factor (BDNF), is also implicated in determining the expression of the serotonin gene. In other words, there is a complex interaction between genes and environment that leads to the development of a depressive illness.

Approximately 40% of the risk of developing depression is due to genetic factors.

Women have a higher incidence of depression and anxiety than men. One of the reasons for it may be explained by the fact that the number of serotonin-binding sites in the brains of women differs from men, and females have a lower level of the protein that transports serotonin back to the nerve cells that secrete it. Some women also demonstrate a difference in their serotonin level in response to changes in hormone levels. This may explain why some women experience greater mood swings and premenstrual syndrome (PMS).

Tryptophan – a naturally occurring amino acid found in the Christmas turkey, bananas, cheese, milk and bread – is a precursor to serotonin. It helps us sleep (hence drinking warm milk at bedtime is a good sleep aid), and might explain why so many of us feel drowsy after Christmas lunch. (It may also have something to do with overindulging in other food and alcohol as well!)

An experiment reducing the level of tryptophan in a group of subjects resulted in the development of depressed moods and impaired learning, especially in those who had a family history of depression.

THE ROLE OF GENES IN DEPRESSION

Sometimes depression can be triggered by stressful life events. However, some people seem to be at higher risk of having this response to such stressors, indicating a possible link to genetics in determining who may be at risk of developing a depressive illness.

People who have experienced a genetic change that is associated with reduced serotonin turnover in the brain were shown to be at higher risk of developing stress-related depressive illness. For example, mothers who have recently given birth may be at risk of post-partum depression.

DOPAMINE, PARKINSON'S DISEASE AND DEPRESSION

Dopamine, another brain neurotransmitter, has been implicated in the development of depression in those with early, negative home environments i.e., where parents have rejected their children. The results of a study examining this suggest that intervention may be useful here in helping prevent depression in this higher-risk group.

Supporters and caretakers can help people suffering from depression by encouraging them to create new life goals for themselves and helping them find their way to success and rewards along the way. This can help boost their natural levels of dopamine and elevate mood.

People with Parkinson's disease have a 50% chance of developing depression as their dopamine levels are severely depleted.

In people with drug addiction, depression is not uncommon and is associated with a lowered level of dopamine D2 receptors in the brain.

People with Parkinson's disease have a 50% chance of developing depression as their dopamine levels are severely depleted.

Treating Parkinson's patients with the commonly prescribed antidepressants that boost serotonin levels has often been ineffective. However, using tricyclics, a different type of antidepressant that affects norepinephrine and serotonin levels in the brain, saw five times the increased chance of seeing improvement in treating the depression.

People with Parkinson's disease are not depressed simply because of the illness they have. The encouraging news is that there are treatments that have been identified that can help such patients with depression as an associated illness.

EXERCISE TO LIFT MOOD

Exercise, such as walking, can have a similar effect to antidepressants in managing depression. This is perhaps partly because exercise boosts the brain's ability to produce new brain cells in the hippocampus, the area of the brain associated with memory and learning. It helps to curtail cortisol levels and boosts natural neurotransmitter production.

Exercise can help in mild to moderate depression and is a great adjunct to include in management of the illness, whether antidepressant medications are being used or not.

When out walking, try keeping your head up so you take in all of your surroundings. When we are feeling low, there is a tendency for us to shut off from external stimuli. We literally don't see what is going on around us. If we have our heads down looking at the ground, lost in our thoughts and avoiding eye contact with others, we are cutting ourselves off from our environment and avoiding social cues from others.

The management of depression after it is diagnosed will often involve consulting a health professional, a G.P., psychologist or a psychiatrist in some cases. Talking through cognitive therapy can also help.

When one is depressed, maintaining normal activities including simply getting up and getting dressed and keeping to a daily routine can make a difference. You can also quickly and easily lift your mood with a little fresh air and exercise, as studies have shown.

Some people will need to take antidepressant medication for a while. They don't work immediately; sometimes the effect is minimal and sometimes there may be side effects. Staying in touch with your health professional is essential to monitor progress, to adjust dosage or tablets and to suggest other therapies as appropriate. Managing depression isn't always easy and it can take many months to resolve. However it can often be helped effectively. The vital thing is to acknowledge that you have a problem, and being able to talk to someone about it is the first step towards recovery.

MOOD FOOD

If we have had a really bad day, sometimes we reach out for comfort food – those foods we indulge in to try and make ourselves feel better. Sadly, after consuming that tub of ice cream or packet of Tim Tams our mood may not be any better. In fact it may be even worse after the sugar and fat hit, combined with the remorse of consuming all those extra kilojoules.

You can, however, improve your mood by choosing certain foods to include in your daily diet.

Brain-healthy foods have been discussed in the section on nutrition.

What you need to remember is that your brain is affected by what you eat, the fluctuations in your blood sugar levels, your level of hydration and your sensitivity to particular foods, additives and preservatives. Additionally, the levels of essential vitamins, minerals, and micronutrients you consume along with carbohydrates, fats and proteins can also impact your brain's overall well-being.

The brain chemicals serotonin and dopamine are made from combining amino acids found in proteins, along with vitamins and minerals.

Because the human brain is predominantly made of fats, we need to include adequate good fat from fish, olive oil and avocados to ensure normal brain function as well.

Skipping meals can lead to low blood sugar or hypoglycaemia. This is associated with an increase in the body's adrenaline levels and an increased risk of anxiety and depression. Plus, vitamin B deficiencies such as folate and B12 have been linked to depression.

For more information about depression and its management contact:

www.beyondblue.org.au

www.actbelongcommit.org.au

Your local G.P. or health provider

SMARTER THINKING: *Anxiety and depression are common disorders in society, which can often be very effectively treated. The crucial step is to seek help early and find which treatment method works the best for you.*

CHANGING YOUR ATTITUDE

"Your attitude, not your aptitude, will determine your altitude."

— Zig Ziglar

What's your attitude? Do you consider yourself a positive person who looks on the bright side of things? Or are you a bit of a pessimist, someone who gets angry at what others have done or said, which you perceive has harmed you in some way? Do you take offence easily or are you someone who likes to look at both sides of an equation, perhaps even asking, "I wonder what's going on in their lives for them to behave or respond in that way?"

Attitude is not something we were born with; it develops and can mould how we look at life, how we respond to life's challenges and how successful we are.

We can choose our attitude, so it is important to choose it wisely.

At the age of 25, Justin Herald was a bit of a no-hoper, broke and in a dead-end job. When challenged by someone who basically told him he would never amount to anything because of his bad attitude, he responded. But his response was to change his attitude. Using $50, he printed some T-shirts with "attitudinal" slogans on them. They sold like hot cakes. Attitude Gear was born and a multi-million-dollar business established.

But for most of us, having a bad attitude will diminish our ability to see or find opportunity in life. It negatively impacts our ability to recover from illness; it may even make a difference in determining how long we live.

Henry Ford said, "If you believe you can or you believe you can't, you are right." In other words, attitude determines outcome on many different levels.

Have you ever experienced the situation where you had the expectation that something might go wrong, and it did? If you go into a test or exam with the expectation that you may not do very well or expect to fail, guess what? It's likely to be a self-fulfilling prophecy.

In contrast, when you have a positive expectation or a worthy mindset, you enjoy the anticipation of something good happening. This gives you a bit of a buzz; you are psyched up and ready to receive your future with positive energy.

One of the key characteristics of those who enjoy long lives is that they have a positive attitude. They look forward to what every new day will bring with a sense of curiosity and anticipated enjoyment.

One long-term study (NECS) looked at 1,500 people in the States who were all over 100 years old. They followed them over 15 years and found that they all embodied an optimistic view on ageing. They did not consider that their actual ages had any bearing on their lives. They remained involved with their families and friends and participated in a variety of activities and new experiences.

This is a reminder that our genes play a role in determining our lifespans, but our environment also plays a very important part in determining our actual longevity.

There are increasing numbers of media reports of older citizens learning how to fly or do a parachute jump. There was a story in our local paper recently about an 87-year-old lady who had just finished her fourth degree.

Of course circumstances are different for all of us. Our life experiences and opportunities may be very different but the way we approach hardship, illness and disease can make a huge difference to how we ultimately survive.

While working in my general practice, I was involved in caring for people with life-threatening illnesses and cancers. I witnessed how they and their families coped and it was inspirational to see how some of them grasped on tightly to life with both hands, deciding to do whatever it took to speed recovery or deal with a terminal illness.

But why wait until a catastrophe happens to make that change? What are the most important things in your life?

Having the latest gadgets, new models of prestige cars and designer clothes may make us feel good in the short term. But it's all just stuff. Having a partner, a family, our health and happiness are usually those ticket items which can't be bought, and yet mean the most to us.

By choosing a positive attitude you can enjoy life more, have a more tolerant and inclusive approach to others, especially those who we perceive as being different. By focussing our attention on what we do have rather than what we don't, our stress levels diminish, and we can experience greater levels of happiness and contentment. With greater happiness and relaxation your mind becomes clearer, emotions are regulated, your thinking is better and you are able to remember more and learn new things.

Emotional regulation is one of the most important life skills we can learn and is usually associated with the highest level of success achieved in life and business.

DEALING WITH BRAIN DRAINERS

Some of us are more adept than others at multi-tasking, juggling distractions, relieving boredom and managing stress, hunger and other demands! Part of becoming more brain fit includes learning ways to prevent these stressors from crushing you.

Many see the integration of work and home life as crucial. We face so many different demands at work and at home it can be a logistical nightmare trying to fit it all together so that it works. Planning is the key.

Does work keeps you away from home longer than you like but there is currently no alternative? Rather than stressing about it, spend your energy working out a way to ensure everyone's needs at home are met. If you are not around to do the housework or shopping, then get someone else to do it. If the kids have sport training after school and it's a struggle to get dinner organised and get them out the door, see if you can share lifts (or even better, share suppers) with another family.

The problem is that once that level of stress builds up to a certain point, it becomes very difficult to see alternatives or find solutions even when they are offered to you. How often do we recognise that we are struggling and yet when someone offers help, we turn it down! This may be because we don't want to be perceived as weak or disorganised. Get over it! Accept help and alleviate some of that pressure. You may be able to return the favour in the future.

RANDOM ACTS OF KINDNESS (RAOK)

Doing something for someone else without any agenda, expectation of acknowledgement or reward makes you feel really good. Imagine if you did something unexpectedly nice for someone else every day, how good would you feel then?

It doesn't have to be something huge or life-changing, either. Have you ever been in a car park looking for change and realise you don't have enough? What impact would it make on your day if a stranger just offered you the money with no expectation of repayment?

It's more than just courtesy, more than simple manners such as opening a door for someone or offering up a seat on a bus. It's about recognising that another human being has a need, which you can help fulfil. That's what makes us human, being able to connect with and help others. Making someone else's day just that little bit better will help improve yours, too.

Have you performed a RAOK today?

Some small gestures you can make:

1. Pay for the order of the person in line behind you at a drive-through window.

2. Put a coin in a parking meter that's about to expire.

3. Smile at someone who looks like they could use one.

4. Say thank you and really mean it.

5. Have a quick chat with an elderly person.

6. Mow the lawn/ rake the leaves of a neighbour.

7. Instead of frowning at a mum with a crying baby, offer to help.

8. Pick up after yourself and your friends when the movie is over.

9. Offer to walk a friend's dog when you go out for a stroll.

10. Pop a funny postcard in the mail to a young niece or nephew.

DEVELOPING AN ATTITUDE OF GRATITUDE

How much do we really need to sustain us and keep us happy? Is it a monetary figure you have in your mind? Is it being able to live in your own home? Is it having enough income to provide for your family?

Our society appears to be focused on striving to have more, to upgrade to a new car, a bigger house, a designer outfit, an overseas holiday. Sometimes we forget just to be grateful for what we do have and this is important for our mental health and well-being.

Keeping a gratitude journal is a very simple yet powerful way of reminding ourselves how much we really have going for us. Each morning or evening, write down five different things you have in your life for which you are grateful. Keep it by your bedside to help you remember to write in it. Consider a nice, proper notebook with a hard cover so it becomes something you can keep and then revisit.

What do you write down? Well, it could be that you are grateful for having a loving partner or healthy kids. You could be grateful that the rain held off for your son's last soccer match or that you got to catch up over coffee with a good friend you hadn't seen for a while.

Reminding ourselves of all the positives in our lives can help us to focus on the bigger picture. So much of the news and media is only negative, and we often dwell too long on what didn't go well for us. If we constantly focus on negative events, we can overlook all the other good things we have enjoyed. Looking at the positives helps us to keep better perspective.

By writing a gratitude journal you may notice a change in your own attitude after a few months. Having an attitude of gratitude helps build mental resilience so when we are faced with a crisis or bad news, we can cope with it more effectively.

BY WRITING A GRATITUDE JOURNAL YOU MAY NOTICE A CHANGE IN YOUR OWN ATTITUDE AFTER A FEW MONTHS. HAVING AN ATTITUDE OF GRATITUDE HELPS BUILD MENTAL RESILIENCE SO WHEN WE ARE FACED WITH A CRISIS OR BAD NEWS, WE CAN COPE WITH IT MORE EFFECTIVELY.

As with any new habit, it takes time to develop. I'm sure there will be some days where you struggle to write down anything you feel grateful for that day. So if the sun rose this morning and you are alive for another day, that is a great start. Keep going, keep writing and little by little you will look forward to acknowledging those five things each day.

LETTING GO

Sometimes we get upset or annoyed by someone's actions or words. If we think they haven't properly apologised or acknowledged the hurt they have caused us, holding onto those feelings can manifest into longer-lasting anger, resentment or hostility. Our perceived sense of wrongdoing by another can affect our ability to function normally, at work or at home.

Letting go is a crucial skill for our mental well-being. This could take the form of telling the offender that you have forgiven him or her or perhaps writing a letter (which may or may not be sent). For example: parents letting go of their hatred and frustration by forgiving the person who killed their child in a motor vehicle accident; or a person getting past feelings of betrayal and forgiving a cheating partner.

This act of forgiveness is not condoning the other person's actions, but allows us to stop living as victims and move on with our lives. We learn to put the experience and hurt behind us and build our emotional intelligence, rather than continuing to ruminate on it and stagnating.

FOCUS ON A BIGGER PURPOSE

It has been reported that people who have a deeply religious faith or a highly developed sense of spirituality are more likely to enjoy a sense of overall well-being and contentment with life. Feeling a sense of purpose for one's life helps connect us to an inner peace and knowledge that what we are doing, learning, and sharing with others is helping them and also helps us develop our own sense of self and legacy.

Studies on longevity have found that people who do live the longest have some similar characteristics, one of which is having a strong sense of faith.

"The better your footprint is, the better it is for all sentient beings."

"The purpose of our lives is to be happy."

— Dalai Lama XIV

That may sound trite or happy-clappy, but choosing to see the positive in life's events and having an optimistic outlook does make it easier to enjoy a more positive life.

This is more than blind optimism or looking through rose-coloured glasses. Yes, there will be times in our lives when bad things happen. However, if we come from a place where we are used to enjoying a balance of positivity and negativity, it is easier to deal effectively with the negatives and not be sent reeling into a place of fear and a downward spiral of more negativity.

Have you noticed that if one person starts out with a negative comment about somebody, then others will join in adding more? It starts in school, but some people never seem to grow out of it. Negative attitudes can spread. Luckily, so too can positive ones.

When the effects of the global financial crisis started to gain momentum, it seemed that every newspaper, magazine and radio station was discussing it and the terrible effects it would have on everyone. Some people responded by simply switching off, choosing to avoid all the negativity by not listening at all.

In the U.K., some of the TV channels run 24-hour coverage of the news, repeating over and over the stories of the day. When my parents came over to visit us in Australia in early 2009, they had been listening to negative media coverage for weeks and had become increasingly fearful and negative in their outlook of the world at large. So we put them on a media diet – simply reducing the amount of total information they could access. (This wasn't too hard as Australian coverage of world events is on a far lower scale compared to its U.K. counterparts.) Gradually their negative outlooks diminished, and they started to look a bit more relaxed and happier.

Totally ignoring the situation isn't helpful either and can contribute to the fear factor. Feeling overwhelmed leads to general depression and an inability to see the positive. It's all about keeping a perspective and being able to look at an argument from both sides, without necessarily having to agree with either.

After the bombings in Bali, people became afraid to travel. It takes time to re-establish trust. However, both the people of Bali and adventurous travellers chose to be positive and move forward and now, just a few years later, Bali is once again booming with many tourists happily returning to vacation at the resorts and hotels. Sometimes you have to move through the fear to get back to a positive state of mind.

If you catch yourself saying negative things about people or events, pause and listen to what you just said. What was the negative comment actually about? Is it because you are expressing your own fears, anxieties, self-doubts and jealousies?

Believing that you can't do something means it is highly likely you will achieve that self-fulfilling prophecy. Having a growth mindset, and allowing yourself the possibility of achieving something that at present may seem impossible, enables your mind to be open to new solutions and greater achievement.

That is the difference when choosing to live with positivity. It leads to possibility.

Having a positive outlook and having the support of your partner or close friends can make a huge difference in the outcome, even when starting from the same place. If we are seeking personal growth, surrounding ourselves with a circle of positive friends to support us, to congratulate us when we have a win, to pick us up when we fall down, enables us to move and develop a more enjoyable, fulfilling and positive life.

When you are happy, you may choose to live a healthier lifestyle, which may also increase your chance of living longer.

SMARTER THINKING: Studies looking at what contributes to longevity have found that many of the people who live the longest are also the happiest. It's not just because of their chronological age; it appears that being happy has a protective effect against illness. It is known that stress and unhappiness can have a negative effect on the body's immune response, making us more susceptible to disease and ill health. The effect of being happy on overall longevity has been compared to that of whether we choose to smoke or not. It's that powerful.

CHAPTER 6

MENTAL CHALLENGE: LEARN SOMETHING NEW

GROW YOUR BRAIN

Our brains love to keep learning. Neuroscience has proven that the human brain is in fact "plastic," meaning it can be moulded or reshaped over the course of time to acquire new information, confirming that we are life-long learners. The word "plastic" comes from the Greek word plastikos meaning "to form."

When I was at medical school (last century!), I was taught that we are born with a finite number of brain cells and that after we reached maturity they started dying off – and we were on the slippery road to mental decline in our dotage. Now we know that far from being finite, we have the capacity to form new brain cells, a process called neurogenesis.

We also used to think that our neural circuits were hardwired and couldn't be changed after childhood. Again not so, the brain's plasticity remains throughout our lives so each brain cell or neuron seeks to form new connections with other brain cells. We have over one hundred billion brain cells and each one can form 10,000 connections or more with other brain cells by forming branch-like projections called dendrites.

FIRE UP BRAIN CELLS WITH NEW CHALLENGES

When we learn something new, brain cells are stimulated and grow new dendrites to form more new connections and strengthen that particular neural pathway or circuit. Our brains are literally jammed full of these multiple interconnecting circuits.

By rehearsing or restimulating these circuits, we continue to strengthen these pathways and build what is termed "cognitive reserve." In a similar fashion, our brains are very clever in dealing with those connections that we don't use or don't serve us anymore by a process called "synaptic pruning."

When two dendrites from adjacent neurons connect, they don't actually physically touch. There is a gap between them called a synapse and the cells pass their messages to each other by the excitatory cell-releasing brain chemicals (or neurotransmitters) into the synaptic space, which are then picked up by receptors on the neighbouring dendrite's tip.

In synaptic pruning, when there is no longer any messaging happening between adjacent neurons, the dendrites actually shrivel and disappear. This means that there is more room to form new connections for the active brain cells. Inactive neurons become tagged or marked out for cell death, a normal physiological occurrence. Obviously we don't want too many dying off too quickly, and so by stimulating the brain to form new connections or form new actual neurons, one develops a brain that is physically more dense. Having a dense network of inter-connecting dendrites is believed to be how we protect our brains from age-related decline. The more we stimulate the brain, the bigger and more robust it becomes.

VARIETY IS KEY

Simply sticking to something you can already do such as crossword puzzles or Sudoku aren't enough. One of the most common questions I get asked is, "Should I be doing crossword puzzles or Sudoku?"

My answer to that is yes, if that interests you and you would enjoy doing it. My caveat, though, is to say that on their own they are not sufficient. Sure they are great for stimulating word recall and verbal fluency and yes, you can challenge yourself to harder versions. But it's all using the same small part of your brain in your speech and language centres, rather than expanding to learn new skills. Rather than just playing cards or bridge, try a variety of different mental stimuli to produce consistent mental challenges.

So think of something that you've always wanted to do. Perhaps you never got round to it, or put it off because of other things taking up your time. Starting up some new hobbies or interests is a sure fire way to stimulate your brain and keep it working at its best.

Have you ever fancied learning Spanish or Japanese, wanted to learn a new style of cooking, take up salsa dancing, join a choir, travel to Peru or learn to play the piano? Then go do. Just pick up the phone and book yourself into that art class you've always wanted to do, the university course you have put off committing to or the swimming lessons that always got put on hold. Your brain will love you for it.

USE IT OR LOSE IT

The common excuses for not doing something are along the lines of "I'm too old," or "my brain's too slow," and they just don't wash anymore. You certainly can keep teaching an old dog new tricks, as many as the old dog wants to take on. True, your speed of processing slows down a bit but by continuing to use your brain you keep it working better. It really is a case of using it or losing it, and once lost, it is much more work to bring it back again.

In any brain fitness program, introducing new mental challenges is the first step. The next is to ensure your brain is challenged by a variety of different stimuli. Some of the best involve several functions at once, such as learning a new dance or sport where motor coordination is involved as well as using our eyes, ears and mental skills. Learning something new stimulates the fresh connections forming between brain cells, and using your body to move adds to that mental stretch, just as if there was a natural progression or challenge.

Similar to children who master the first grade of piano and then move onto the second and then the third, the brain's mental stimulation continues when it gets to stretch and work in novel situations. Once we've mastered something, we no longer get that same boost for our brains. Having a variety of mental challenges and interests is useful so there is never time for the brain to get bored.

And do choose something you enjoy doing. Often we don't know if we'll like the new activity we've signed up for. Simply, if you don't, then stop! Move on and choose something different. You needn't be a world champion or an Olympian. Just have a willingness to try something and if you love it, chances are you'll get better and better at it. Having fun helps motivate us to continue, boosts self-confidence and increases one's skills.

So look around and explore new classes and options – which brain activity most suits your interests and your lifestyle?

SMARTER THINKING: *The key with mental challenge is to find:*

- *Something new to challenge those brain cells*
- *Variety to stretch our brain cells*
- *A range or continuing challenge in the selected activities*

Learning is neuro-protective and we are life-long learners.

CUT OUT THE NOISE

Working from home has many varied blessings. One of which is the peace and quiet, allowing thoughts to flow … except when renovations are underway.

While living through a home renovation, my mind was subjected to the additional external stimuli of loud banging, power-saws, the radio playing at full blast and some fruity conversational interactions between the tradies starting at 6:45 a.m. each morning.

Was this distracting? Yes! Did it impact my ability to concentrate and focus on the task at hand? Yes!

Noise is a form of stress and stress is bad news for our mental fitness and our brains. When you hear a sudden loud or unexpected noise such as a car back-firing or a police siren, you may respond with a startle reflex. The body and mind is quickly alerted to the possibility of danger and the need to get out of the way. This is the classic fight-or-flight response.

The noise itself, apart from making you jump, does no real long-term harm.

Noise is a form of stress and stress is bad news for our mental fitness and our brains.

WHAT IS THE IMPACT OF CHRONIC, LOW-LEVEL NOISE?

It is actually low-level ambient noise that does the most harm in terms of affecting one's ability to think clearly and retain information, not jack hammers and rock concerts, which can cause actual hearing loss. The danger is in the background noise that comes from living in congested cities with loud, constant road traffic, the sound of sirens, school playgrounds and living under the flight path of aeroplanes.

And although we think we get used to it and take little notice, unfortunately the effect on the brain continues and it does not truly adapt.

In this case, the body experiences ongoing stress, inducing cortisol release. Ongoing cortisol secretion impacts the brain by killing off brain cells (never a good thing), and reduces our brain cells' ability to form new connections with each other. In particular, it impairs the prefrontal cortex, the area of the brain used for executive decisions, planning and organisation; and is thought to reduce dopamine levels to that area as well. Dopamine is a neurotransmitter important for regulating the transmission of information from other parts of the brain to the prefrontal cortex.

The National Institute for Occupational Health and Safety in the United States has reported that ambient noise affects people's health generally by increasing stress levels. Additionally, the American Census has rated noise a higher problem than crime, litter, traffic or inefficient government.

NOISE AFFECTS YOUR ABILITY TO FUNCTION

In the workplace, low-level noise from working in open plan offices has been shown to lead to higher levels of stress and lower task motivation.

In one study, 40 experienced female clerical officers (average age, 37 years) were assigned to either a quiet office or one with low-intensity noise. Those working in the noisier areas experienced high levels of stress hormone (measured in urinary epinephrine levels), made 40% fewer attempts to solve an unsolvable puzzle and made only half as many ergonomic adjustments to their work stations. In other words, their brains were stressed so they were less willing or able to participate as well in work tasks, compared to those in the quieter work areas.

And it's not just adults in the workplace who may be disadvantaged from trying to work in noisy environments.

An Austrian study demonstrated how low-level noise induced a stress level response (with raised heart rates and blood pressure) in children and could lead to an impaired ability to learn. They looked at 115 kids in Grade Four. Half lived in quiet areas (sound level equivalent to 50 decibels), while the other half lived in noisier areas.

The study showed that children subjected to chronic noise stress were more likely to demonstrate "learned helplessness," a condition linked to poverty and some forms of depression. They simply don't bother to make the effort to try. Girls seem particularly at risk.

So, maybe we need to be aware of the ambient noise that surrounds us and our families on a day-to-day basis. Especially now that we understand it is a potential cause for limited thinking capacity.

Are there any ways you can implement changes in your own workplace or at home to minimise the effect of ambient low-level noise and assist your brain function?

Encourage your work place to implement changes that enable staff and workers to work more easily in a quiet environment.

SMARTER THINKING: Noise is a distraction that can impair our ability to think well. In modern life we are surrounded by a cacophony of noises, which can literally make it impossible for our brains to find that quiet space where we can simply think.

AVOID MULTI-TASKING

We are all time-poor, with multiple demands on our busy schedules every day.

There is so much more to do in our lives than just a full time job or running a business. We have to include all the extras – making time for family and friends, running the kids to and from school, sporting activities, shopping – and our to-do lists seem never-ending. There is always something else waiting, pending, or demanding our attention.

So how do we cope?

We end up devising our own strategies to manage, and the tempting thing is to multi-task. Women in particular seem to try to multi-task more often than men. We are even encouraged to do it. I've seen job advertisements stating that potential applicants must be good at multi-tasking.

It feels good to tick all those items off the list. We congratulate ourselves on our ability to cook the dinner while speaking to our mother on the phone, supervising the kids' homework and flicking through that long work document that has to be read and edited before an all-important meeting tomorrow morning.

Okay, confession time. Who has sat in a meeting or listened to a talk while your mind has wandered off and you surreptitiously check your emails, or send a text message or tweet on your phone? Then all of a sudden you realise you have missed a critical statement or piece of information. Or even worse – you are asked to comment, which is a bit hard because you weren't following the line of conversation. Oops.

Unfortunately your brain lets you down. It has a design flaw.

The area of the brain that is involved in "executive" thinking for planning and organising, called the prefrontal cortex, takes up only a small part of our frontal lobes. It can handle one task exceptionally well. Give it two or three and the brain goes into overdrive by switching attention quickly between the different tasks it is trying to deal with. That's why attempting to text or use your mobile phone while driving is so dangerous. Besides the obvious error of taking your eyes off the road, there is literally a gap of attention when your brain is frantically switching quickly from one task to the other. It is in those small fractions of seconds that disaster can occur.

Our brains can usually only pay attention to one thing at a time. There are occasions when we are multi-tasking but it's for things that don't actually require our full attention, such as walking and talking. But if you are reading a book and someone comes along and strikes up a conversation with you, which task can your brain deal with then? Answer: the one it chooses, but not both.

DO ONE THING WELL

The biggest challenge is to resist the temptation to multi-task in the first place. When you notice that you are attempting several things at once, remind yourself that your brain doesn't like it. It's exhausting (for the brain) and unproductive.

Don't scatter your focus. Use a methodical approach:

- Organise your to-do list with the top "must do" three or four items for the day.
- Prioritise in the order you will tackle them.
- Allocate your full attention to each task and do not start the next one until the first is completed.

Studies have shown that by following these few simple ground rules we will complete all the allocated tasks in a shorter period of time using less brain energy and effort, and with fewer errors.

Sounds like a no-brainer to me.

 **SMARTER THINKING:** *Multi-tasking is exhausting for our brains. Give your brain a break by prioritising your tasks, starting with the most important first. Don't move on to the next until the first is finished. You will make fewer mistakes and get finished more quickly so you have more time to spend on other activities such as time with your family.*

COGNITIVE TRAINING

Brain training, does it work? The short answer is yes, but it is important to understand what brain training actually is. It is not merely playing brain activity games, which, while fun and help you to improve in that particular brain function, does not produce long-lasting cognitive change. Crossword puzzles and Sudoku are great mental activities but they only challenge a small portion of the brain. The principle of brain training is that it does produce long-lasting improvements in brain function that change by providing a variety of challenging exercises leading to brain change.

Brain-training software and online programs are designed to assess and enhance our cognitive abilities. If looking to trial one, it is important to ask yourself a few questions first:

- Does this product have any scientific back up or peer review to support its claims of effectiveness?

- Does it allow you to work out which areas of brain function you may wish to focus on and which program will suit you the best?

- Does it provide an assessment and feedback on your progress?

- Is it designed to steadily challenge your skills as you progress?

- Do the games or programs look user-friendly and something you would be happy to work at on a regular basis?

- Are you prepared to spend the required time and effort to get the most out of the program? If you don't enjoy computer work then perhaps you might be better suited to look for alternative mental stimulation.

The principle of brain training is that, by providing a variety of challenging exercises that lead to physiological brain change, it can produce positive long-lasting improvements in brain function.

If choosing to follow a brain-training program means you would be giving up socialising activities or leaving your home, then perhaps you would be better off keeping in touch with friends and family.

Cognitive or brain training is effective. Scientific evidence is now available showing that memory training does produce positive brain change, even in those with mild cognitive impairment.

We are already seeing the introduction of brain-training programs into schools, especially to assist those kids with certain learning disabilities.

They have been introduced into the sporting arena to help athletes focus, and as driving programs to keep both seniors and young drivers safer on our roads. Of course they are essential as brain fitness and memory enhancers for people looking to improve their cognitive skills, particularly as they get older.

In America, some physical fitness gyms are starting to put in brain-training programs to allow people to get a physical and mental workout all in one place.

SMARTER THINKING: Brain-training programs that can provide lasting cognitive improvement are becoming more readily available. It isn't necessarily for everyone, so choosing a program is always an individual choice. Training requires persistence and ongoing challenges to produce the desired outcome; it's far more than just playing brain games.

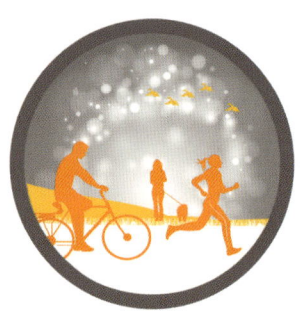

CHAPTER 7

EXERCISE AND BRAIN HEALTH: GET MOVING

HEALTHY BODY, HEALTHY BRAIN

One of the factors in maintaining good brain health is regular physical exercise. We've heard the message that keeping fit is good for our hearts, our waistlines and our general well-being. Now there's an added component. Research and many studies have repeatedly documented that physical exercise is good for our brains as well, for two reasons.

Exercise promotes neurogenesis, the brain's ability to produce brain cells. But even more than that, exercise provides the right environment in the brain to allow these baby brain cells to survive, mature and become integrated into our existing neural pathways. We are literally growing our brains.

Second, exercise promotes existing neurons or brain cells to form more connections between each other. This allows stronger neural pathways to be established and enhances memory and learning.

As we get older we become aware that our thinking reaction times become slower and we are less adept at planning and multi-tasking. It's harder to take in and remember new information. Our ability to concentrate and focus diminishes and we may even notice early symptoms of neurodegenerative disease. Yikes!

Does the thought of donning lycra, straining muscles and getting really sweaty (or being in the close vicinity to someone else in lycra who is sweaty) put off any desire to exercise?

Well the good news is you don't have to.

The fundamental requirement is regular exercise, and it can be as simple as increasing the amount of walking you do and looking for opportunities to increase your incidental exercise activity.

Which exercise you choose boils down to personal choice and what is most appropriate for you, your age and personal medical health. It can be walking, swimming, running, golfing or cycling; whatever you like and are happy to do on a regular basis. It can even include going to the gym (lycra not essential).

HOW CAN I INCREASE MY ACTIVITY LEVELS?

Are you stuck at a desk all day in front of a computer screen? The first thing is to get up and off your bottom. Try planning a 10-minute break each hour where you get up, have a bit of a stretch and move around the office. Better still, try to get outside into the fresh air.

It's like long-distance flying. After sitting for too long in an aircraft we know it's good to get up and have a stretch.

When parking your car, rather than spending time trying desperately to get the closest spot to the entrance, try parking a little further away from your destination so that you have to walk that incremental distance.

> It's like long-distance flying. After sitting for too long in an aircraft we know it's good to get up and have a stretch.

In the choice between the elevator or the stairs, take the stairs. Well, maybe not if it is the 18th floor, but how many times do we see people waiting patiently for the lift, just to take them up one or two levels? Our bodies were designed to move and walk. Our ancestors walked many miles each day. Now with all the modern conveniences of cars, lifts and travelators, our legs may only carry us from the house to the garage and back each day.

Get a dog! They are always ready for a walk and will provide the necessary incentive with a wag of the tail, fetching the lead (or even the trainers) and of course, looking at you with those big, brown pleading eyes. They don't care if it's cold, dark or raining. If the offer is a walk they will always want to go.

IS IT EVER TOO LATE TO START EXERCISING?

Absolutely not. And obviously, the earlier, the better. Kids who participate in sport at school tend to do better academically and be better adjusted in terms of mood.

The aim is to participate in some form of regular activity that we enjoy throughout our lives. Be consistent. We need to make exercise part of our everyday lives, part of our daily routine that we simply do, without excuses.

You are never too old to start exercising to enjoy the brain benefits.

A resistance exercise program was introduced into a frail-aged facility in the United States and the outcome was so positive that the program has been adopted more widely. Those residents that participated in a 10-week program saw improved muscle strength, increased walking speed, better cognition and memory, and enjoyed an improved sense of well-being. Pretty impressive!

 **SMARTER THINKING:** *Exercising is an activity we can enjoy across our entire lifespan. Increasing your level of physical activity is a natural part of helping your body and mind to stay in top condition.*

BENEFITS OF EXERCISE FOR THE BRAIN

STUDIES HAVE SHOWN THAT JUST GOING FOR A WALK EVERY DAY FOR 20 MINUTES SIGNIFICANTLY ADDS TO OUR OVERALL WELLBEING AND REDUCES THE RISK OF STROKE BY 57%.

Walking three times a week for 30 minutes each diminishes the risk of developing dementia (by 10% at least). A study carried out at UWA in 2008 showed that just this moderate exercise in a group of over 50-year-olds with some memory problems produced improved cognition and memory over a six-month period, which was then maintained after the study finished. An American group found that people who exercise at least three times a week, whether it be walking, swimming or jogging, can reduce their dementia risk by over 30%. This reduction in risk also holds true for those at higher risk of Alzheimer's and vascular dementia.

Walking that bit further is even better, with improved benefits for every additional kilometre walked. Participating regularly in exercise lifts your mood and sense of well-being, reducing the likelihood of depression and improving cardiovascular fitness.

If you are feeling a bit stressed, under the pump or have a problem, going for a walk can help you gain clarity in your thoughts and enable you to resolve these issues as well as improve your attitude. Studies show that exercise has a similar effect to antidepressant medication in helping manage depression, through the production of new brain cells.

As one get older, the area of the brain associated with memory and learning, the hippocampus, starts to shrink. This coincides with a gradual decline in cognitive ability and memory. Exercising helps to maintain and increase the size of the hippocampus. The bigger it is, the better your ability to retain spatial memory (to keep learning) and to retain memories.

When we exercise, the amount of blood flow to the brain increases, and the brain receives more oxygen and glucose. Regular activity promotes the formation of new blood vessels in the brain, producing greater energy and giving our existing brain cells a better chance of survival. Even better, studies indicate that regular exercise enhances neurogenesis – the production of new brain cells in the hippocampus – and is particularly important for learning and memory.

And yes, there is more.

Better than a free offer of extra steak knives, exercise stimulates the increased production of substances called BDNFs, which are crucial to supporting and nourishing existing brain cells.

Those who exercise more show less loss of grey matter, which means greater retention of the executive functions of the frontal lobes for better concentration, attention and planning.

Plus, it appears that exercise can induce a change in the expression pattern of a wide array of genes. This is particularly important, for example, when someone is carrying a gene that may put him or her at increased risk of developing a condition like Alzheimer's disease. If that gene is not expressed or if the expression is delayed, it could have a significant impact in reducing or delaying the probability of developing the disease.

SHOULD WE BE DOING AEROBIC OR RESISTANCE TRAINING?

The answer is both.

Aerobic exercise is the cornerstone to improving brain fitness. Having said that, strength or resistance training is also vital.

When you exercise aerobically you get your heart rate up, which is good for the heart, pumping more oxygen to your brain and making your lungs work harder too.

As we age, our muscle strength starts to decrease naturally. By working with weights, exercise machines and resistant, elastic training bands (the thick ones used by personal trainers and physiotherapists) we can work the muscles to keep them strong, enabling us to keep doing things in our daily lives that we take for granted. This strength or resistance training helps us maintain a better sense of balance, increased flexibility and muscle endurance.

WHICH IS THE BEST FORM OF PHYSICAL ACTIVITY FOR THE BRAIN?

The best physical activity is the one that gets your heart rate up, is something you enjoy doing and is something you can incorporate easily into daily routine. You're not limited. Do something new, try a variety of different challenges and find something that will continue to be a challenge as it gets more difficult. It's exactly the same in physical exercise for the brain. The best activities or workouts require us to learn something new, varied and challenging, as a dance routine in a Zumba class requires mental and physical input because we have to integrate physical coordination along with memory (what step comes next?) and hopefully, a sense of rhythm.

WHEN IS THE BEST TIME TO EXERCISE?

That depends on your individual routine and what works best for you. It's better to do the exercise when you know you have the best chance of "finding that thirty." Many people like to exercise in the morning and certainly research suggests that being physically active before going to work refreshes you and prepares you to cope better with the day's demands. Your brain is better able to take in new information and manage demanding situations.

But that isn't going to work for everyone, and certainly a number of people find they enjoy exercise at the end of the day to help them unwind.

Getting started:

- Set a date to begin and a goal for what you expect to achieve in the first week, or month. Even if the goal is just to get out for 10 minutes every day, that's an excellent starter objective.

- Choose an exercise buddy who will help you to keep going with your new routine.

- Tie up your shoes, walk out the front door, and keep walking. It can be that simple.

- Keep safe. If the only exercise you have done over the last few years is to walk to and from your car, then start slow and build up gradually. That will help increase your endurance and enjoyment and keep you from injuring yourself.

- Follow a program initially with a timetable to help you keep to your new routine.

If it doesn't always happen and life gets in the way, don't use that as an excuse to give up. Persevere, persevere, and persevere. Gradually you will find you look forward to your daily exercise as you experience the rewards of clearer thinking and improved overall fitness and health.

Professor Leon Flicker from the Western Australian Centre for Health and Ageing has reported that lifestyle changes including physical activity have the benefit of warding off Alzheimer's as well as heart disease.

Now where did I put my trainers?

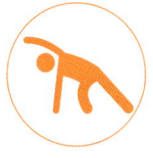

SMARTER THINKING: The bottom line is that participating regularly in physical activity has clear benefits in maintaining good brain health and improving cognitive function. The benefits are fairly broad and help us perform better in tasks requiring a higher level of executive functioning such as planning, working memory, and coping with distractions.

EXERCISE CAN HELP MANAGE OTHER RISK FACTORS

Any doctor (including me) will tell you that exercise can do a world of good for many ills. These include health issues that also have an impact on your brain fitness. For that reason we'll look at them individually as they become more epidemic in Australian and world populations.

These risk factors contribute to poor brain health and are avoidable:

- Obesity
- Type 2 diabetes
- Smoking
- High cholesterol
- Hypertension

OBESITY

There has been an exponential increase in the number of people around the world who are obese and have diabetes, both risk factors for dementia.

MIND YOUR WEIGHT

For many, the battle of the bulge is seemingly the result of consuming too much fat, being too sedentary or simply eating too much. As you get older your metabolic rate declines, so while you still experience hunger and enjoy your food you need to reduce your total food intake to keep your weight in the normal range.

Being overweight or obese also puts you at risk of other chronic illness and disease. You increase the risk of cardiovascular disease, stroke, diabetes and cancer. But there is something else to be aware of as well.

Being overweight or obese doubles your risk of developing dementia or Alzheimer's disease. It is associated with having a smaller brain volume and this affects brain function in specific areas:

- In the hippocampus, the area specialised for learning and memory
- In the frontal lobes, the executive suite, which is concerned with planning, organisation and being able to pay attention
- In the anterior cingulate gyrus, an area involved in decision-making, empathy and emotion
- In the thalamus, an area associated with coordinating other brain areas

A SPECIAL AREA OF CONCERN: WAIST SIZE

It is actually belly fat that puts people most at risk. Having a big tummy with stick legs and arms puts us at greater risk than someone who is more generally rounded or hour-glass shaped, i.e., an apple vs. pear shape. The implication here is that you don't have to be particularly overweight to be at increased risk, if all the extra weight is sitting around your middle.

Being obese in middle age, having an elevated systolic blood pressure (that's the top reading of your blood pressure) and having high total cholesterol are all significant risk factors for dementia on their own, and individually can double your relative risk of dementia. Put them together and you can end up with six times the risk of dementia. So we really need to watch that those love handles don't sneak up on us.

One study performed as part of the Framingham Heart Study (in Massachusetts, U.S.A.) had over 700 subjects. The mean age of the group was 60 years and 70% were women. The study looked at the associations between Body Mass Index (BMI), waist circumference, waist-to-hip ratio, CT-measured abdominal fat and MRI studies of the subjects' brains; looking at total brain volume and the number of brain infarcts (mini areas of stroke) present. The results showed a strong correlation between central obesity (abdominal fat) and the risk of developing dementia and Alzheimer's disease.

A meta-analysis of 10 international studies covering a 10-year period confirmed these findings, revealing that obesity increases the relative risk of dementia for men and women overall by an average of 42% compared to people of normal weight.

However, after the age of 65, it appears the trend is reversed. Annette Fitzpatrick from the University of Seattle reported on the results of her study that observed nearly 300 people without dementia. At age 50, subjects had their weight and height recorded, and then repeated measurements at age 65 to calculate the BMIs at the different ages.

Over a five-year follow up, subjects classified as obese (BMI >30) were more likely to have developed dementia. However the older subjects who were underweight (BMI <20) also had an increased risk of dementia, and the older, fatter subjects appeared to have gained a protective effect in later life.

So there appears to be an obesity paradox. There is a change in the predictive ability of BMI with dementia risk with age. Why?

IT IS ACTUALLY BELLY FAT THAT PUTS PEOPLE MOST AT RISK. HAVING A BIG TUMMY WITH STICK LEGS AND ARMS PUTS US AT GREATER RISK THAN SOMEONE WHO IS MORE GENERALLY ROUNDED OR HOURGLASS SHAPED, I.E., AN APPLE VS. PEAR SHAPE.

This is not yet fully understood. It has been suggested that weight loss in older life may precede the onset of dementia. Studies have shown that women in particular will show weight loss about 10 years before the first signs of dementia become apparent.

The easiest solution is preventative. Maintain or get to a normal weight at your current age. Pay special attention to reducing abdominal fat. By combatting obesity you can reduce your risk of developing dementia or Alzheimer's later on.

A GROWING RISK GROUP: OBESE TEENAGERS

The burgeoning incidence of obesity and diabetes in young people is frightening. Teens are at increased risk of cardiovascular disease, cancer and premature death due to their poor eating habits and inactive lifestyles. Of those that survive these issues, they also remain at far greater risk of cognitive impairment and dementia as obese and/or diabetic adults.

A new study shows that obese kids with Type 2 diabetes reveals some brain abnormalities, and on mental testing shows reduced cognitive performance. These kids will likely function less well academically. Previously, studies that found these brain abnormalities on MRI scans in older subjects with diabetes had attributed them to vascular disease rather than the effect of diabetes itself on the brain.

The study looked at a group of 18 obese adolescents with Type 2 diabetes and another group of similarly obese adolescents who hadn't yet developed significant insulin resistance or Type 2 diabetes. Both study groups came from similar socio-economic backgrounds and ethnicity.

They were asked to complete some mental tests. The results of the group with diabetes were significantly lower in the areas of memory, spelling and overall academic function. They also showed white matter abnormalities on brain scans. This is the first time that cognitive deficits have shown up in this age group as a consequence of the combination of obesity and diabetes.

The results highlight the urgent need to address both obesity and diabetes. More and larger studies need to be undertaken to verify these findings and to get support from government and health professionals so effective health programs can be developed

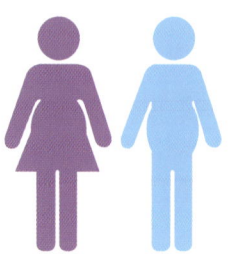

WE HAVE YET TO COUNT THE IMPACT OF YOUNGER PEOPLE ALREADY BURDENED WITH THE SIGNIFICANT HEALTH IMPAIRMENTS OF OBESITY AND DIABETES THAT WILL ADD TO THIS TOLL.

and implemented to deal with this tide of obesity and diabetes. The challenge is to help kids already diagnosed with insulin resistance to improve their insulin sensitivity through weight management, healthy eating and exercise.

By failing to address the issues of overall inactivity, obesity and diabetes, we are adding to the already significant social and economic burdens that increasing rates of dementia will have on us over the next few decades.

It won't be just the baby boomers who are at risk of dementia simply because of their increasing ages. We have yet to count the impact of younger people already burdened with the significant health impairments of obesity and diabetes that will add to this toll.

SMARTER THINKING: Obesity is a modern disease linked to a higher risk of premature death, cancer, heart disease and dementia. It is likely that the future generations, by remaining obese, will live shorter lives. Keeping your weight in the healthy range, eating a balanced, brain-healthy diet and getting enough physical exercise are critical. and getting enough physical exercise are critical.

TYPE 2 DIABETES

Statisticians say western societies are facing a tsunami of people developing dementia and Alzheimer's over the next couple of decades. This is associated with our ageing populations; we are all living longer, so our relative risk of developing dementia rises as well.

Doctors are concerned that we seem to be ignoring the fact that people living with Type 2 diabetes and obesity will dramatically increase the future diagnoses of dementia.

Both diabetes and obesity are known risk factors for dementia.

Adults who develop diabetes before the age of 65 have twice the risk of developing dementia compared to non-diabetics and they also have an increased risk of depression.

Doctors are concerned that we seem to be ignoring the fact that people living with Type 2 diabetes and obesity may have a higher risk of dementia.

But it is our children that worry me the most. Twenty years ago the number of kids diagnosed with Type 2 diabetes was in the order of 2%. It was an extremely rare condition. Now 30% to 50% of all those diagnosed with Type 2 diabetes are between the ages of 9 and 19. Those in their 30s have seen a 70% increase in diagnoses.

The scary thing also is that there are an even greater number of people with undiagnosed diabetes in the general population.

WHAT IS TYPE 2 DIABETES?

When you eat a meal, the carbohydrates in it are broken down and released into your blood stream as sugar, leading to an increase in your blood sugar level. This then stimulates the pancreas gland to release insulin hormone which works to restore the blood sugar level back to normal, by sending the glucose to tissues that need it for energy or for storage.

If the body is repeatedly overloaded with excess glucose, the body's ability to respond to the insulin is diminished, leading to a condition called insulin resistance. Increasing amounts of insulin then get produced, but it can no longer exert its effect. This leads to the condition of Type 2 diabetes where blood sugar levels are consistently too high and associated with elevated insulin levels.

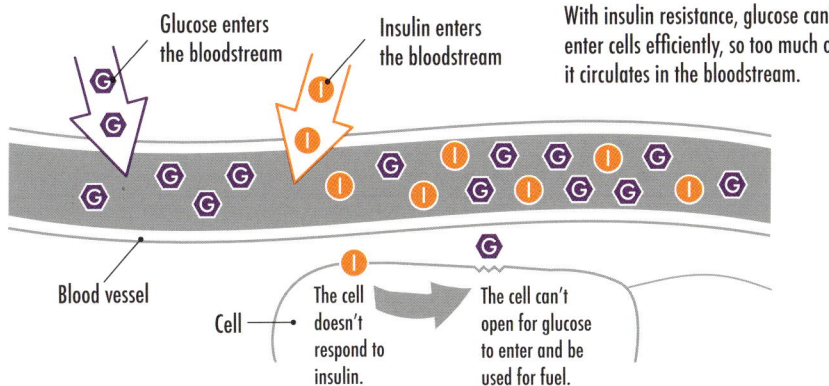

Glucose enters the bloodstream

Insulin enters the bloodstream

With insulin resistance, glucose can't enter cells efficiently, so too much of it circulates in the bloodstream.

Blood vessel

Cell

The cell doesn't respond to insulin.

The cell can't open for glucose to enter and be used for fuel.

This distinguishes it from Type 1 diabetes where the specialised glands in the pancreas are unable to produce insulin.

DIABETES CAN AFFECT YOUR MENTAL FITNESS

If you have diabetes, you have a higher risk of cognitive decline and dementia.

In a study of 2,300 older women aged 70 to 78, non-diabetics scored twice as high as diabetics on mental testing. It was also found that the longer the person had diabetes, the more poorly she performed.

In another multi-ethnic, multi-centre study of 10,000 people, the results of cognitive tests taken six years apart were compared. In the age group of 40- to 70-year-olds, diabetes was again linked to greater cognitive decline.

WHAT DOES DIABETES DO TO THE BODY AND BRAIN?

Diabetes affects multiple organs in the body including the blood vessels, heart, eyes, brain and kidneys and is insidious in how it gradually erodes cognitive ability. Elevated blood sugar levels contribute to hardening of the arteries (atherosclerosis), which increases the risk of heart disease and stroke. In the brain, this vascular damage is linked to an increase in small infarcts (injury to small arterioles in the brain) or tiny strokes. Having persistently elevated blood sugar contributes to brain atrophy, cognitive impairment and damage of brain cells. The loss of brain cells is especially prominent in the area of the hippocampus, affecting memory and learning. Diabetic patients who have developed diabetic retinopathy can have twice the risk of developing cognitive impairment.

The excess insulin also contributes to brain damage. The brain has its own insulin receptors. Having higher levels of insulin has been linked to increased levels of amyloid, the protein associated with plaques found in Alzheimer's. Having excess insulin also plays a role in stimulating inflammation and in reducing the levels of acetylcholine – the brain's essential neurotransmitter for memory.

But it's not just diabetics who are at risk of impaired brain function and reduced mental performance. It has been shown that even drinking a sugary glucose drink will adversely affect your ability to perform memory tests. So the key is to avoid big swings in blood sugar levels.

Because we know that diabetes is associated with an increased risk of cognitive impairment and dementia, it is even more important to consider your lifestyle and dietary choices.

Simple choices can make big differences.

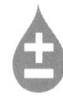 **Keep blood sugar levels in the normal range**

 Maintain a healthy body weight

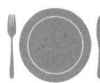 **Eat a nutritious and brain-healthy diet low in saturated fat**

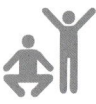 **Exercise for 30 minutes a day (moderate intensity)**

 **SMARTER THINKING:** *Diabetes paired with obesity are two of the most prevalent and dangerous modern day diseases facing society. Type 2 diabetes can often be prevented by keeping your weight healthy, eating a healthy, balanced diet and getting enough exercise.*

SMOKING

Okay, hands up. Who doesn't know that smoking is bad for your health and is associated with an increased risk of heart disease, stroke and cancer?

Apart from remote tribespeople such as those living in the Envira region of the Brazilian/Peruvian rainforest, most people are aware of the negative effects cigarettes have on their health.

But did you know the damaging effect smoking has on your brain? And did you know about the damage you can inflict on your kids' brains by subjecting them to second-hand smoke?

Let's start with the proven evidence as it relates specifically to the brain. Smokers have:

- reduced capacity for memory
- reduced problem-solving skills
- increased risk of dementia

Of course this doesn't begin to cover the array of cancers and diseases smoking can cause, or the socially negative aspect of having one's clothes and hair smelling like smoke.

In the 10 seconds it takes for the nicotine and other chemicals to reach your brain after the first drag on the cigarette, changes occur in the brain affecting mood, well-being and memory.

Thought that smoking makes you more alert? Think again. A U.S. study by the University of Michigan revealed that smokers have a slower and less accurate thinking ability. Long-term smoking damages your memory, your ability to problem-solve and reduces your I.Q. Ouch!

WHY DOES SMOKING GIVE YOU A "BUZZ"?

In the brain, acetylcholine is a neurotransmitter associated with a number of the body's functions including learning and memory. It also facilitates other neurotransmitters that are associated with mood, memory and appetite. The nicotine attaches to the acetylcholine receptors in the brain, mimicking its actions and promoting dopamine levels.

Dopamine is the brain chemical associated with experiencing pleasurable feelings. Ever wondered why some people say they enjoy smoking? It could be the raised dopamine levels talking. Elevated dopamine partially answers why it is so hard to stop smoking, as the nicotine addiction wants you to keep those nice dopamine levels up.

MORE BAD NEWS

If you smoke, you will score lower on memory tests. Period.

Smoking more than a packet a day will lead to increased difficulty remembering names and faces. And remembering names is one of the most commonly-voiced concerns about memory loss.

Smoking more than a packet a day provides a regular cocktail of toxins including toluene (also found in paint thinners and solvents – and we know what that does for your brain), which can cause confusion and memory loss.

Ladies, those of you who smoke into middle age and menopause need to be aware that nicotine lowers your blood oestrogen levels and may inhibit the effect oestrogen has on your brain, exacerbating any brain cell effects of the fluctuating oestrogen levels. Women who smoke score 20% lower in tests of executive thinking i.e., reasoning, planning and organising.

WHAT IS THE LATEST EVIDENCE?

Dr. Markus Richards at University College, London, conducted a study on 5,362 people born in 1946 and divided them into groups of smokers, non-smokers and ex-smokers.

They were given a list of 15 words for two seconds each and were then asked to write down as many as they could remember. In the second part of the test they were shown a page of letters and they were given one minute to find and remove all of the P's and W's.

The results showed the smokers had the lowest scores for memory. Those who had given up smoking had a lower level of decline than those who had continued to smoke. So if you do smoke you will still be doing your brain a huge favour by stopping.

The relationship between memory and smoking was most marked in those who smoked 20 or more cigarettes a day. In other words, the more you smoke, the worse the effect on your memory.

Smoking can therefore accelerate age-related memory problems. Is this surprising? Well, impaired memory is not uncommon in smoking-related illnesses such as cancer, heart disease, stroke, bronchitis, emphysema and asthma. Why smoking has this effect remains unclear but it could be because smoking increases a person's risk of developing high blood pressure (itself a risk factor for dementia). Or it may be that smoking has an effect on the supply of oxygen on the brain. Another possibility is that it could be a direct toxic effect of the multitude of toxins found in cigarette smoke. Whatever the underlying reasons, it is clear that smoking affects memory and is a risk factor for dementia.

Hint: this is a <u>really</u> good reason to give up the smokes.

The benefit of stopping now is that there is less memory deficit the earlier you quit. And it's never too late to stop.

If you smoke, you have an addiction (as well as a shrinking brain) so it takes a decision, commitment and perseverance. It's not easy. But you can do it.

PASSIVE SMOKING, DIABETES AND DEMENTIA RISK

Let's look at the impact that passive smoking has on our brains and those of our children. Passive smoking is associated with an increased risk for developing impaired glucose intolerance, a precursor for diabetes that is itself a risk factor for dementia.

A U.S. study on 4,500 subjects followed over a 15-year period, showed the following results in percentages of those who developed impaired glucose tolerance.

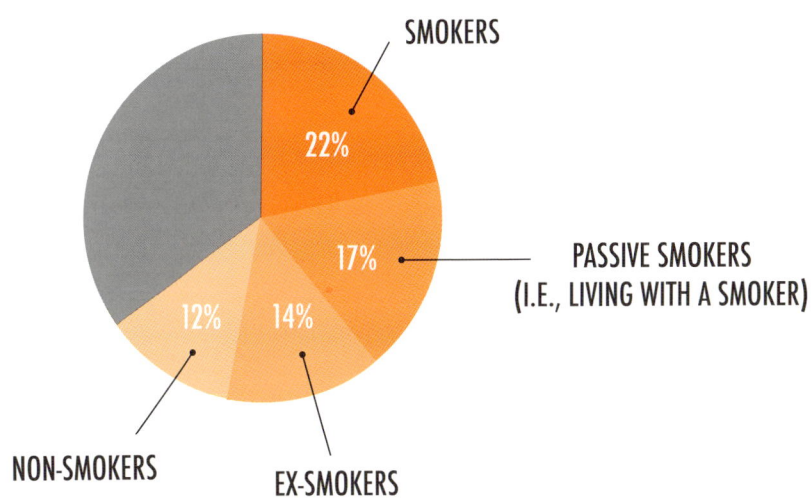

In other words, the passive smoking group had a higher risk of developing impaired glucose tolerance even when compared to the ex-smokers. And smokers themselves had almost twice the risk of non-smokers. Yet another valid reason to give up the habit.

We are witnessing an explosion in the number of people with obesity and diabetes, both major risk factors for impaired cognitive performance and dementia.

Why add that risk to those around you, especially the children you love, by continuing to smoke?

Passive smoking (second-hand smoke) can lead to:

- cancer in non-smokers
- the development of heart disease in non-smokers
- an increased risk of impaired glucose metabolism (a precursor for diabetes) in non-smokers

Heart disease and diabetes are both risk factors for dementia.

In the February 2009 edition of the British Medical Journal, it was stated that, "second hand smoke (i.e., passive smoking) increases a person's risk of dementia and other forms of cognitive impairment and also is associated with poorer cognitive performance in children and adolescents."

Good grief. If ever there was an incentive to give up smoking for the sake of your kids, surely this has to be a big one!

The message is stark. Passive smoking increases your risk of dementia.

DUMB OR DUMBER? SMOKING CAN LOWER YOUR I.Q.

Smoking also reduces academic performance in younger children and adolescents.

Dr. Mark Eisner for the University of California agreed in his statement that the evidence is emerging: parental smoking may impair a child's cognitive development. Prolonged exposure to passive smoking can lead to cardiovascular disease, increased risk of stroke and cognitive decline.

If you've noticed that I am repeating the message, it is because I think it is crucial to understand this.

Still in the U.S., a study by Leslie Jacobsen at Yale revealed that adolescents who smoke showed inaccuracies and impairments of their working memory. It was even suggested that teenagers who smoke are perhaps going to need additional educational support because of this.

Boys (who tend to start smoking earlier than girls) were found to be most impaired in tests of selective and divided attention. This was highlighted further by a study just published by Professor Weiser of the Tel Aviv University Dept. of Psychiatry and Sheba Medical Centre at Tel Hashomer Hospital.

In this study, 20,000 healthy young men aged between 18 and 21 who had enlisted in the Israeli army were asked about their smoking history and underwent intelligence tests. Around 28% reported they smoked one or more cigarettes a day, 3% were ex-smokers and 68% were non-smokers.

The results of the intelligence tests showed the average I.Q. for the non-smokers was 101, the average for the smoking group was 94, and those who smoked a packet or more a day scored even lower at 90.

In an average population of healthy young men an I.Q. score would normally be expected to lie between 84 and 116. In this group, socio-economic background was not a factor. These were all healthy young adults from a variety of backgrounds. Interestingly, in twin brothers where one was a smoker and the other was not, the non-smoking twin on average registered a higher I.Q. The only difference for the skew in results was that the smokers were consistently lower in their I.Q. scores.

If we don't want our kids to be dumbed down, then we seriously need to encourage them not to take up smoking in the first place as well as seeking to minimise any potential exposure to passive smoking.

SMARTER THINKING: As parents we all want the best for our kids and to see them grow and succeed in life. Why would we knowingly diminish their ability to do well academically, by either smoking ourselves or allowing them to take up smoking as teenagers? Remember, passive smoking is as deadly as smoking itself. If you are an adult who smokes, giving it up will not only benefit your health, it will also benefit the health of your family in many ways, including protecting their brain fitness.

CHOLESTEROL AND THE BRAIN

The link of excess cholesterol to heart disease has been around for many years. You may have been encouraged to have your cholesterol levels checked by your GP at some stage, particularly if you have a family history of heart disease. We need cholesterol for a number of vital biochemical pathways, so cholesterol in itself isn't the problem. The real problem is that our western diets have led us to consume too much fat and the wrong type of fat.

There is an important link as well between cholesterol and the brain. But before looking at the implications of cholesterol and cognitive skills, let's pause for a moment and quickly look at how our bodies deal with cholesterol.

The human body has developed two pathways to deal with cholesterol. In the first, our dietary source of cholesterol (from foods containing animal fat such as meat and cheese) is absorbed from the gut and transported to the liver. Here, some of the cholesterol is sent up to the gall bladder along with some bile salts to help us digest other fats further along in the gut. This cholesterol is then either reabsorbed, completing a recycling loop, or is excreted from the body. In the second pathway, cholesterol is repackaged in the liver into the type called VLDL and sent out via the blood where it is converted again – this time into LDL or "bad" cholesterol and sent out to all other cells, where it is used to form a part of every cell membrane. The body has a built-in regulator (via receptors in the liver and the cells themselves), to monitor LDL levels and determine how much cholesterol is released in this way. Once finished with the cells, the cholesterol is repackaged once more into HDL, the "good" cholesterol, to either be reabsorbed and reused or broken down and excreted.

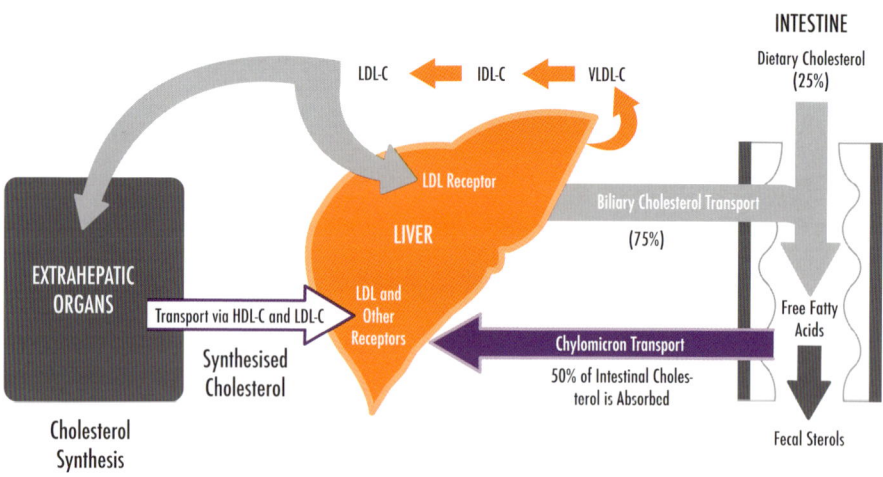

So, the body has an excellent self-regulatory system in place to keep our cholesterol levels normal.

The problem is that dietary changes in western society have seen us adopt a far greater intake of saturated fat, leading to an intake of dietary cholesterol that the system wasn't designed to cope with. This leads to the excess cholesterol in our blood vessels, forming plaques and causing inflammation. That can lead to narrowing of the arteries, and the clinical manifestation of heart disease in the form of angina or heart attack.

Because we have become more aware of the need to modify our diets and consume less fat, and drugs called statins have been introduced to help us to lower blood cholesterol, there has been a reduction in the level of heart disease in the community.

THE BRAIN MAKES ITS OWN

The brain makes its own cholesterol through specialised cells called astrocytes. It gets moved to our brain cells by transporter molecules called apolipoprotein E (APOE). Aha! Do you remember the link between the gene for APOE and the risk of dementia?

The plot thickens. These APOE molecules enable our brain cells to take up the cholesterol and insert it as specialised rafts of lipid within the cell membrane.

That's right, your brain makes its own cholesterol that it uses to form synapses (the connections between brain cells). It is also used to form the vesicles or storage structures located at the synapse that contain the neurotransmitters, the brain's chemicals that are passed from one brain cell to the next. We have a "fat" head and it is essential the brain can produce sufficient cholesterol for healthy brain function. Having too little cholesterol in the brain is associated with Alzheimer's disease and other neurodegenerative conditions.

THE CONFUSING DISASSOCIATION OF BRAIN CHOLESTEROL AND BODY CHOLESTEROL

Having a high blood cholesterol level in midlife is a known risk factor for Alzheimer's and people who receive treatment with statins appeared to lower that relative risk.

Statins are drugs used to lower blood cholesterol by inhibiting an enzyme required for its production. Enzyme inhibitors were thought to potentially reduce cholesterol levels and become the wonder drug that might reduce the risk of Alzheimer's, but this proved not to be the case.

In mice studies it was initially demonstrated that the statin drugs could reduce cellular cholesterol and be linked to a lower production of beta amyloid, but follow-up trials failed to demonstrate the expected result that statins would prove useful as a preventative for Alzheimer's disease.

In a study of 6,000 people with high cholesterol who received either a statin or placebo, no difference in the rate of development or dementia in either group was found over a three-year period. To add to the confusion, studies on the brains of people with Alzheimer's disease revealed that these people often had lower levels of cholesterol in the brain cells membranes, compared to their healthy counterparts. So the statins might actually be doing our brains a disservice, because the brain cholesterol is vital to form synapses, which are essential for normal brain cell communication.

Part of the issue here is that there is a disassociation between the level of cholesterol measured in our peripheral blood circulation, and brain cholesterol levels.

Statin treatment has been shown to reduce the amount of circulating amyloid in our cerebrospinal fluid by up to 40% and yet there was no difference in dementia rates. Beta amyloid has been described as being the "baddy" in Alzheimer's, based on the pathology findings of the brains of Alzheimer's patients.

THE DISPARITY OF AMYLOID DEPOSITS AND ALZHEIMER'S DISEASE

It has been recognised for some time that some people with clinically advanced Alzheimer's show no pathology of beta amyloid plaques in their brains and, conversely, people with apparently no cognitive loss were found to have brains riddled with amyloid plaques and neurofibrillary tangles.

This was one of the findings from the Nun study. This is an ongoing study that began in 1986 following the lives of 678 members of the School Sisters of Notre Dame religious congregation. Initially this study examined the contributing factors that allowed many of the sisters to enjoy great longevity. It subsequently developed into a much larger study into the ageing process. Each of the participants also agreed to donate her brain for research at death.

In the study, the nuns underwent rigorous mental and physical tests each year. The researchers also had access to meticulously kept records of each nun's background and upbringing. Examining the brains after death, the researchers found a curious paradox. The clinical symptoms of dementia demonstrated by the sisters did not necessarily match the expected pathological findings. In other words, the brains of some nuns with diagnosed clinical Alzheimer's disease were "clean" of amyloid, whilst others with no apparent sign of any cognitive impairment had brains that were full of it.

This did not match the expected finding and placed large question marks over the theory that Alzheimer's disease was a result of the amyloid and neurofibrillary tangle build-up. Current thinking is that Alzheimer's may be actually a disease of the synapse. Where synaptic connections are lost, brain functions of memory and thinking become affected and gradually lost.

The role of the synapse and brain cholesterol levels may be more intimately entwined

Current thinking is that Alzheimer's may be actually a disease of the synapse.

than had been previously realised. Some scientists now believe that beta amyloid could actually be evidence of the brain trying to protect itself from metabolic damage.

Cholesterol has been shown to be crucial for proper synapse functioning. Adding cholesterol to a petri dish full of neurons or brain cells will stimulate new synapses to form. So it follows that having less brain cholesterol is associated with reduced brain function.

However, peripheral cholesterol levels (i.e., measured in the body) have been shown in studies to produce adverse effects on brain function. Chronic high levels of cholesterol in rat studies have been shown to impair memory and increase inflammation. High levels were also associated with increased formation of beta amyloid and tau protein, as well as micro bleeds, all of which resemble the pathology associated with Alzheimer's disease. It is possible that multiple mild micro-vascular bleeds in the brain, silent strokes, and mild blood brain barrier damage contribute to the resultant Alzheimer's disease.

Cholesterol on its own is not the only culprit for causing Alzheimer's, but it appears to have a clear role in the development of the disease.

HIGH CHOLESTEROL WITH DIABETES REQUIRES EXCELLENT GLYCAEMIC CONTROL

Diabetes is a recognised risk factor for dementia. It is also associated with a higher risk of depression and eating disorders. What has now been found is that diabetes affects how much cholesterol our brains can make.

Studies using mice with type 1 (insulin deficient) diabetes looked at gene expression in an area of the brain called the hypothalamus. It was found that in these mice, gene expression for the production of cholesterol was reduced. Treating them using insulin reversed the problem.

They also found that those mice that were unable to make brain cholesterol gained more weight and ate more, indicating that diabetes may affect those brain hormones associated with appetite regulation.

This finding adds to our understanding of the relationship between diabetes, cholesterol and healthy brain function. If you have diabetes, having tight glycaemic (sugar) control and maintaining a healthy weight are essential to help your overall brain health and to protect against future cognitive decline.

CAN YOU DO ANYTHING ABOUT YOUR HIGH CHOLESTEROL LEVEL?

The answer is yes. A study from Temple University looked at how changing diet, even in early-to-moderate Alzheimer's disease, could make a difference in slowing down the rate of cognitive impairment.

To reduce your cholesterol consumption, try reducing the amount of processed meats such as salami and sausages, and pies, pastries and biscuits. Trim excess fat off meats and watch your cheese and dairy consumption. Bake, grill, stir-fry or steam food rather than deep frying.

Cut down on foods rich in methionine, which are broken down to homocysteine in the body. Homocysteine is a recognised risk factor for dementia. By eating fewer foods high in methionine (such as red meat, fish, beans, eggs, lentils, onions, yoghurt and seeds), Studies on rodents were able to demonstrate that mice fed a high methionine diet leading to cognitive decline had this cognitive decline reversed by cutting out the methionine from their diet.

But, you may ask, these foods high in methionine are also good for us, aren't they? Yes, it simply comes down to the quality and balance of our diets.

SMARTER THINKING: Cholesterol in excess is a risk factor for dementia. Managing your cholesterol level by diet, exercise, and statins if required, will help to reduce that relative risk. Our brains still need some cholesterol, which it produces naturally itself to allow normal synaptic communication.

HYPERTENSION

I was sitting in my G.P.'s office recently, being told something I didn't want to hear. My blood pressure was too high and I needed to start medication with antihypertensives.

I didn't want to have to take medication. I had always planned on not being on anything apart from fish oil and glucosamine supplements until I was at least 90 years old. I consider myself fit. I exercise daily, my weight is normal, I eat healthily, I don't smoke and I keep an eye on how much wine I drink each week.

But my family history includes hypertension and stroke on both my mother's and father's side. And I do recall a conversation with my obstetrician who was managing my pregnancy-induced hypertension a number of years ago. He said, "Jenny, you are likely to develop hypertension as you get older." Harrumph. I heard, but didn't want to listen. But who am I trying to kid?

I have what is called "essential hypertension." The cause is as yet unknown.

I don't like it. But I can deal with it and take my pills. The reason why? Simple: I value my brain cells too highly to ignore the problem. As a doctor, my medical training has taught me the consequences of untreated hypertension.

KEEP YOUR BLOOD PRESSURE NORMAL

Hypertension has been described as a silent killer. You can't feel if your blood pressure is too high. We rely on readings taken with a sphygmanometer to get an accurate idea of the state of our blood vessels.

The blood pressure reading essentially tells us the peak or systolic pressure our hearts have to exert with each contraction to pump the blood around our bodies. The lower reading or diastolic pressure gives the resting pressure of the circulatory system in between heartbeats.

If the readings are too high, we run the increased risk over a period of time of blood vessel rupture that causes a stroke or cerebrovascular accident. Other organs are affected as well, including the kidney, eye and heart. None of which is good news.

WHAT IS THE EFFECT OF HIGH BLOOD PRESSURE ON MEMORY AND COGNITION?

Studies have shown that having high blood pressure can contribute to memory loss and other declines in brain function in people over 45.

In one study of over 19,000 participants aged 45 or older, they found that with each 10-point increase in diastolic pressure, the risk of cognitive difficulty increases by seven points.

BUT HOW HIGH IS HIGH?

We need to keep our diastolic pressure (the lower of the two readings, indicating the pressure of the arterial system at rest) at below 90mmHg.

With 25% to 30% of the Australian adult population having high blood pressure, I am clearly not alone. For the vast majority of people like myself, we have "essential hypertension" where no specific cause is identified. However, having high blood pressure causes problems by causing our arterial walls to thicken and lose their elasticity, leading to reduced blood flow and tissue death.

Having reduced blood flow to your brain becomes an issue especially during times when you need it to work harder. For example, when you want to pay attention or work out a solution to a problem. The decrease of available blood flow to your brain leads to fewer brain cells being activated, and leads to an increased number of memory lapses.

In older people, having high blood pressure can predict who is at risk of developing impaired executive function (organising, planning and decision making) and who may be at a greater risk of progressing to dementia. One study of 900 octogenarians showed that high blood pressure was associated with an increased risk of developing dementia when frontal lobe functioning was impaired.

Because stroke and transient ischaemic attack (TIA), or mini-strokes are leading causes of risk of cerebrovascular disability followed by dementia, controlling hypertension is a simple and effective way to potentially reduce the incidence of forecasted dementia in this group significantly.

WHY CUTTING THE SALT CAN HELP YOUR BRAIN

We all need some salt in our diets for normal health; around six grams per day. But as with so many other factors in the western diet, it's when we have too much that can lead to significant health issues, any many of us eat far too much salt in our daily diets. The problem with salt is that in excess it can lead to high blood pressure. Having high blood pressure puts more stress on your kidneys, your heart and your blood vessels – putting you at increased risk of stroke and vascular dementia.

The other problem with salt is that it gets into our food by stealth. You may be conscious of the need not to add salt to cooking or at the table. However, 80% of the salt we consume is hidden. It's present in many processed foods and unless we read the labels, we don't know it is there. Common culprits include chips, savoury snack foods and biscuits, soups, and sauces. But what about baked beans, processed meats, canned foods in brine (salt water) and fast foods such as pizza?

Other than refraining from adding salt to food and reading labels, what else can you do to reduce your salt intake?

There are low-sodium salt alternatives. These are often based on potassium chloride. If however, you are already on antihypertensive medication, some of these drugs include a warning about not taking potassium supplements in any form. If in doubt, check with your doctor or local pharmacist to make sure this is a safe alternative.

Use alternatives to give extra flavour to your food. Try using lemon juice, pepper, onion, garlic, chilli, or vinegar to give your meals some extra zing without the salt.

So it's essential to diagnose and treat hypertension in midlife to protect you from developing cognitive impairment further down the track.

If you are over 45 and haven't had your blood pressure checked for a while, now would be a good time to make an appointment and get it checked by your G.P.

If it is too high then some simple lifestyle changes could help:

- Keep your weight in the healthy range
- Don't smoke
- Reduce your alcohol consumption
- Do some regular exercise
- Keep your cholesterol in the normal range
- Eat less saturated fat
- Use less salt in your diet

Hypertension has no symptoms, but is easily managed and keeping it in the normal range could make a big difference in helping you save your brain.

SMARTER THINKING: Having a history of high blood pressure that remains untreated is associated with a higher risk of cognitive decline and dementia. Getting your blood pressure checked is easy to do. If your blood pressure is too high then lowering it through healthy brain lifestyle choices and medication as necessary will help protect your brain.

CHAPTER 8

YOUR NAME GAME PLAN

By now you may realise that building brain fitness is not just something nice to have, it's essential to optimise your own individual brain health so you can enjoy the results of better thinking today and the potential for healthy brain function in the future.

While it's good to look at what we can do to protect our brains from Alzheimer's disease and other forms of dementia, brain fitness is about enjoying optimal brain health and function at any age; to think well, to remember more and enjoy clarity of thought even when under pressure. This means incorporating those strategies for greater emotional resilience, enhancing our coping skills and bouncing back when things go awry.

Increasing brain fitness for our children promotes better learning, and boosts their chances to achieve greater success in all areas of their lives academically, emotionally and socially.

Brain-fit adults are better able to deal with potentially overwhelming issues, like having too much to do in too little time. They are more resilient to those stressors which, left unchecked, could lead to poor performance and mental distress, or even mental illness.

For older adults, baby-boomers and seniors, the potential for early or undue deterioration of the brain exists. This is real – it happens and is happening – to many of us. But, the question is how do you know if it will happen to you? For some aspects of brain disorders, there are known indicators to suggest relative risk, but generally we won't know until it's too late.

There are many simple, practical things we can all easily do to improve our chances of living longer with a healthy brain. They are not fool-proof, but there is plenty of evidence to suggest that making careful choices about nutrition, cultivating a positive attitude, continuing to challenge our brains and engaging in physical exercise can make a significant difference.

So, we have a choice: be pro-active and do things that will increase our chances of staying a bright spark longer, or go with the flow. What's it to be?

Surely it's a no-brainer? It's as easy as remembering your **NAME**®!

Initiating and achieving positive change for improved brain function and health is something everyone is capable of doing, if we so choose. That's what Santiago Ramon y Cajal, neuroscientist and Nobel Prize winner for medicine, said at the turn of the 20th century, many, many years before the concept of neuroplasticity became known and accepted.

Knowing what is possible and having the information to build better brain fitness is a great first step.

But the second step is committing to the process of increasing your level of brain fitness and taking the necessary actions to implement a more brain-healthy lifestyle.

What happens then depends on the actions you take to determine your own program, strengthening your new brain-healthy habits in relation to Nutrition, Attitude and stress management, Mental challenge and Exercise. Remember it is all in the **NAME**®!

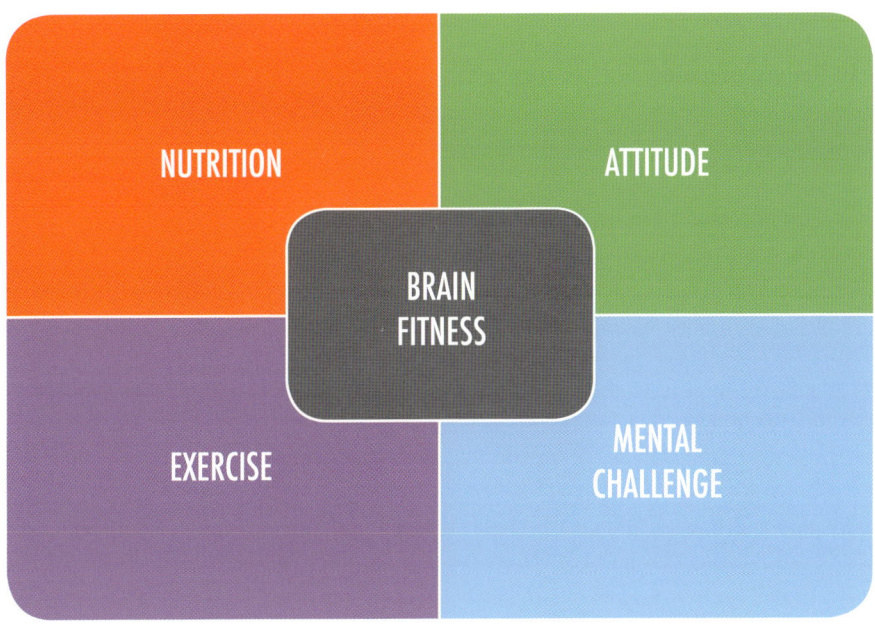

For your own Brain Fitness Plan, go to *www.drjennybrockis.com/plan* and download your complimentary "30 Day Brain Fitness Plan."

Tips To Help You to Implement Your Own Brain Fitness Plan:

Identify the areas within **NAME**® that you feel need improvement.

NUTRITION

Aim to eat oily fish 2-3 times a week.

Look for ways to include a variety of fruits and vegetables, especially the highly coloured varieties, at every meal.

Ideally, a meal should comprise one-third each of vegetables, protein and carbohydrate.

Add some seeds and nuts to provide antioxidants and good oils.

Use olive oil for your salads.

Where possible, include fresh rather than processed foods into your diet. Preparing meals using fresh ingredients often takes no longer than some of the pre-prepared items and tastes so much better.

Drink plenty of water: 6 - 8 glasses a day.

Rather than making radical changes to your diet or excluding unhealthy foods entirely, aim to make small, gradual changes by adding in healthy alternatives whenever possible, allowing your palate to get used to the differences. Denying yourself the foods you enjoy is a recipe for failure. You may find it possible to resist temptation initially, but most people find that old habits will creep back in.

Try eating new healthy foods that you haven't had before. You will probably find that as you start to eat more healthily, you'll feel better and more energised, which is a powerful motivator to continue eating those new foods.

Be more mindful in the way that you eat. Slow down, notice what you put into your mouth, savour the flavours, the texture and the enjoyment that good food brings. If you eat fast food, do the same thing. By becoming more aware of what goes into your mouth, you will start to appreciate what you do or don't like about particular foods.

Encourage other family members to sit down together for meals. Turn the TV off and focus more on each other's company and the food being shared. Teaching your children and other family members to cook is a great life skill, and has recently been enhanced by all the cooking reality TV shows popular now.

ATTITUDE

Attitude is always going to be a choice. If you notice that you are grumpy or reacting strongly to a particular person or comment, that awareness is the first step towards choosing a different response.

If you are quick to lose your temper, you may be under considerable stress. Try to identify those triggers causing you to respond in this way. If stress is an issue, how can you modify the impact it is having on your brain and your thinking?

Try to identify things that bring you joy and happiness. Is there a way you can engender more of those "feel good" moments? Notice how your tone of voice and the way you speak to others influences how they speak to you. Choosing to be more tolerant, accepting and understanding of others will often result being treated more fairly and kindly in return. That's a win-win situation, which your brain loves! It reduces stress and promotes a greater sense of well-being and happiness.

Are you keeping a gratitude journal? Every day, morning or night, think of five things you can be grateful for; it could be the fact it was a beautiful sunny day, or that you are healthy, or that you are in a loving relationship, or that you spoke to a friend you had lost touch with, or received a compliment, a bonus or completed a challenging task. Whether it is big or small, all these items accumulate in your gratitude bank and like other forms of saving, it pays dividends. The more you practise being grateful, the more you will appreciate the good things around you. They were always there, but in our busy and often negative world we just forget to see them.

Practise smiling and saying hello. Emotion is contagious. If you smile at a person, they are likely to smile back, which makes you both feel good. Sharing a smile can set someone else up to be more positive in their day as well as yours. Having a more positive mood makes it easier to learn, to innovate and to complete your tasks.

Stay social. Our ability to relate, connect and bond with other human beings contributes to what makes us human. Spending time with family and friends is a great way to stimulate your brain, to promote well-being and joie de vivre (literally, joy of life). Studies have shown that those who live the longest are often people who remain curious and engaged with the world around them.

With modern technology it's possible to be in contact with virtually anyone on the planet. So reach out and connect with others by telephone, Skype, SMS, email, snail mail and best of all, face to face.

Stress is a useful survival tool. You need enough to get out of bed in the morning and fired up for the next challenge or project. As with many aspects of our brain, it is all about maintaining balance. Insufficient stress can lead to boredom. Too much can impair prefrontal cortex function and lead to memory and learning problems, especially if cortisol levels become too high and toxic.

Learning a variety of stress management tools and practising them regularly enables you to manage those stressful situations more easily and become less agitated by them. If dealing with difficult clients or family members is an issue, learning techniques of deep breathing, meditation and mindfulness can help to keep things in perspective. So the next time there is an argument looming, you have the strategies in place to minimise the threat response in your brain and calm down.

Mindfulness meditation, yoga, pilates, tai chi and other forms of exercise are all fabulous ways to lower your stress and feel more mentally alert.

MENTAL CHALLENGE

Your brain is constantly busy, responding and adapting to all the sensory input it receives. Because it is plastic, your brain has the capacity to be a life-longer learner, to adapt in many instances to injury it may receive, and to allow you to rewire some neural circuits to develop new, useful habits and supersede the old ones.

Challenging your brain requires three things:

☐ Something new that it hasn't experienced before

☐ Something with variety to stretch your mental muscle

☐ Something with continuing challenge

The mental challenge can be further divided into low tech and high tech.

Low-tech challenges include activities that you may already be practising. However they remain important as a means to help build and maintain cognitive reserve.

Include some stimulating mental activities on a regular basis.

If you are at work, you could spend 10 - 15 minutes during a break to do a crossword or read an article, a newspaper or a chapter in a book.

At home you could look for a way to have 30 minutes of focussed attention daily, playing a card game or board game with others.

If you have been to a recent movie or concert, discuss the experience with others and recount the highlights.

Sign up for a class in a subject that interests you or a hobby you have always wanted to try.

High-tech challenges include brain-training software programs that are readily available. There is a wide range for different budgets and tastes. So have a go, experiment with a couple and see which ones you enjoy the most. Many have a free trial period so you get a chance to experience what the program offers.

The best programs are those that are designed by people in the neuroscience or neuropsychology field with specific areas of brain function that can be worked on such as working memory, visual-spatial awareness and attention skills. These programs can be quite demanding. Beyond having the ability to use a computer, it is important to check that you can see your progress and improvement, and perhaps even get feedback on your progress.

EXERCISE

What is interesting about the research on exercise and brain function is the consistency of the findings. Bottom line, we all need to exercise regularly (minimum of thirty minutes a day, preferably more), lifestyle and individual situation permitting.

The other interesting thing to note is that exercise not only stimulates healthy brain function, it works synergistically with other components for brain fitness. For example, brain training is great for stimulation for better memory and cognition. However, teamed with regular exercise, the results are even better. The same applies to exercise and stress management, and exercise and nutrition.

In other words, exercise is very important in all aspects of brain health. So whatever it takes, get moving.

One of the biggest concerns is the amount of the time we are spend sitting. For many people, their workday consists of sitting in front of a computer screen, which is shown to be detrimental to physical and brain health. Many organisations are starting to recognise this and incorporating strategies to stop people sitting so much.

If you spend more than a few hours sitting each day, then look for opportunities to get up and move.

- ☐ Try standing while answering a phone call or when you take a break from your work and are perhaps checking your social media sites.

- ☐ Instead of sitting on a chair, try a fit-ball, which requires the body to use a variety of different muscles to keep you upright.

- ☐ Have stand-up meetings.

- ☐ Invest in a treadmill desk.

- ☐ Use your computer's clock as a prompt to get up and take a five-minute stretch.

There are lots of things you can do, it's just a matter of remembering to do them, and often.

Exercise doesn't need to be high intensity for your brain to benefit but it does need to be sufficient to get your heart rate up and to make you slightly puffed. The main thing is to start and be consistent. Use whatever it takes to develop the habit of physical activity every day.

If you have not been exercising regularly before, start slow and build up. If you start too enthusiastically and do too much, you run the risk of injury, which could stymie your chances of building a new exercise habit. If you are over 50, check with your doctor first to ensure your chosen program is appropriate for your age and fitness level.

Many gymnasiums offer a personal assessment to provide a tailored program to your needs. They are often inexpensive and well worth the investment. If gyms and equipment are not your thing, then simply getting out for a daily walk is a great start.

Remember your exercise routine, like mental challenge, needs variety and on-going challenge. Add some weight training, stretching and flexibility exercises, which have proven benefits to enhance brain function.

Choose something you will enjoy and have fun. After all, who wants to do something on a regular basis that they don't like? Me neither. So it's time to get out there, start moving and build that brain.

There are other aspects that contribute to brain fitness, including adequate sleep and managing your physical health. The bonus section for your brain fitness plan is to ensure that you get a good night's sleep of 6-8 hours and to address those modifiable risk factors which may impact your brain health. It's time to find out:

- ☐ Is your weight in the healthy range? Just because global obesity is on the rise, doesn't mean it is acceptable or prudent to allow yourself to be overweight. Obesity is a risk factor for reduced cognition and dementia.

- ☐ Do you have Type 2 diabetes? If so, it is crucial to keep tight control of your blood sugars to minimise the potential risk of dementia.

- ☐ What's your cholesterol level? It's important to get it checked for your heart health and your brain health too.

- ☐ Do you know your blood pressure? High blood pressure often has no symptoms. Unchecked, it can increase your risk of vascular dementia and stroke.

- ☐ Are you a smoker? Give it up. Smoking is toxic to your body and brain. So do yourself and your family a favour and quit.

THE BOTTOM LINE

My goal with this book is to provide a framework of knowledge and practical steps that anyone can use to take better care of his or her brain.

It's a serious opportunity that can have serious consequences if not grasped. Making some simple, practical and sustained changes to our current life habits can make a real, positive difference.

Be aware of how your brain works and what you can do to look after it as best you possibly can!

If having read this book, you do nothing other than ask yourself – now what is it that **NAME**® stands for? – That would be a good start. Just remember your **NAME**® – please!

As Hippocrates wrote:

"If we could give every individual the right amount of nourishment and exercise, not too little and not too much, we would have found the safest way to health."

NEXT STEPS

If you have enjoyed Brain Fit! you may be wondering what else you can do to build up your own level of brain fitness and smarter thinking.

Becoming brain fit provides the foundation for optimal brain health and function, allowing you to work more effectively in those areas that could be holding you back. In addition, developing better communication skills, improved interpersonal relationships and greater resilience is the easiest way to enjoy greater well-being, happiness and fulfilment.

You can visit www.drjennybrockis.com and

- Access over 250 articles on Dr. Jenny's blog relating to our brain's function and performance.
- Download some extra resources to help you embed your new brain healthy habits including a thirty day planner and brain fitness infographic at www. drjennybrockis.com/fitnessplanner
- If you need a little help to get started, why not sign up for Dr. Jenny's free 5-day Procrastination e-course.
- Sign up to Dr. Jenny's weekly e-newsletter that contains cutting edge news and insights for better brain function and performance.
- Book to attend one of Dr. Jenny's keynote presentations or workshops.

Jenny is passionate about helping individuals and organisations achieve their best outcomes through better brain health and function. She is an educator, mentor, author and award-winning speaker. She seeks to inspire greater performance, by simplifying the complexity of brain science into practical applications that are relevant to everyday life.

Her mission is to make brain fitness as much a part our culture as physical fitness.

A life-long learner, she is a qualified "Nightingale" nurse from St. Thomas' Hospital, holds an M.B. ChB. (Brist) F.R.A.C.G.P. (WA), and has completed a post graduate certificate in the Neuroscience of Leadership.

After successfully setting up and running her own Group Medical Practice for many years Jenny decided to focus on speaking, writing and authoring and now works primarily with corporates and the workplace sharing her knowledge and expertise to inspire, motivate and activate the brains of others.

Happily married with two young adult children, Jenny lives in beautiful Perth, Western Australia, with two Border Terriers and one dog-weary cat.

She loves to spend time with her family and friends, enjoys travel, exploring Australia's rugged Outback, snow skiing, (although there is never enough snow in Western Australia), and is addicted to books and learning. To find out more or to get in touch, visit www.drjennybrockis.com

Brain Fit! Is her first book.

BIBLIOGRAPHY

Recommended further reading

N. Doidge. The Brain that Changes Itself: Stories of Personal Triumph from the Frontiers of Brain Science. 2007, New York: Viking.

J.J Ratey and E. Hagerman. Spark: The Revolutionary New Science of Exercise and the Brain. 1st edn. 2008, New York; Little, Brown.

J. Medina. Brain Rules: 12 Principles for Surviving and Thriving at Work, Home and School. 2009, Seattle; Pear Press.

J. Bolte Taylor. My Stroke of Insight. 2008, London; Hodder & Stoughton.

D. Snowdon. Aging with Grace: The Nun Study and How We Can All Live Longer, Healthier and More Vital Lives. 2001, London. Harper Collins.

S. Halpern. Can't Remember What I Forgot: Your Memory, Your Mind, Your Future. 2008, Three Rivers Press.

R.M. Sapolsky, Why Zebras Don't Get Ulcers. 3rd edn. 2004, New York: Times Books.

REFERENCES

GENERAL

World Alzheimer Report 2010. www.alz.co/uk/worldreport

Access Economics Reports. Caring places: Planning for Aged Care and Dementia 2010-2050

Dementia: a public heath priority. World Health Organisation 2012

Deloitte Access Economics. **Dementia Across Australia: 2011 - 2050**. 2011. Alzheimer's Australia; Canberra. Available at http://www.fightdementia.org.au. Accessed 31st October 2012.

D.E. Barnes and K. Yaffe. **The projected effect of risk factor reduction on Alzheimer's disease prevalence.** Lancet. Neurology, 2011. 10 (9) :819-828

ANXIETY

G. P. Shumyatsky, E. Tsvetkov, G. Malleret, S. Vronskaya, M . Hatton, L. Hampton, et al. **Identification of a Signaling Network in Lateral Nucleus of Amygdala Important for Inhibiting Memory Specifically Related to Learned Fear.** Cell - 13 December 2002 (Vol. 111, Issue 6, pp. 905-918).

ATTENTION

Daniel Smilek, Jonathan S.A. Carriere, J. Allan Cheyne. **Out of Mind, Out of Sight: Eye Blinking as Indicator and Embodiment of Mind Wandering**. Psychological Science, 2010; DOI: 10.1177/0956797610368063.

Kalina Christoff, Alan M. Gordon, Jonathan Smallwood, Rachelle Smith and Jonathan W. Schooler. **Experience Sampling During fMRI Reveals Default Network and Executive System Contributions to Mind Wandering**. Proceedings of the National Academy of Sciences, 2009; DOI: 10.1073/pnas.0900234106.

Peter F. Delaney, Lili Sahakyan, Colleen M. Kelley and Carissa A. Zimmerman. **Remembering to Forget: The Amnesic Effect of Daydreaming. Psychological Science**, July 2010; vol. 21, 7: pp. 1036-1042.

BERRIES

Krikorian, et al. **Blueberry Supplementation Improves Memory in Older Adults.** Journal of Agricultural and Food Chemistry, 2010; 100104141245097 DOI: 10.1021/jf9029332.

BRAIN TRAINING

E. De Villers-Sidani, L. Alzghoul, X. Zhou, K.L. Simpson, R.C.S. Lin, and M.M. Merzenich. **Recovery of Functional and Structural Age-related Changes in the Rat Primary Auditory Cortex with Operant Training.** Proceedings of the National Academy of University of Virginia (2009, March 20).

Papp, et al. **Immediate and Delayed Effects of Cognitive Interventions in Healthy Elderly: A Review of Current Literature and Future Directions**. Alzheimer's and Dementia, 2009; 5 (1): 50 DOI: 10.1016/j.jalz.2008.10.008.

CHOCOLATE

Martin, et al. **Metabolic Effects of Dark Chocolate Consumption on Energy, Gut Microbiota, and Stress-Related Metabolism in Free-Living Subjects.** Journal of Proteome Research, 2009; 091007113151065 DOI: 10.1021/pr900607v.

Karin Ried, Thomas Sullivan, Peter Fakler, Oliver R. Frank and Nigel P. Stocks. **Does Chocolate Reduce Blood Pressure?** A Meta-Analysis. BMC Medicine, 2010; DOI: 10.1186/1741-7015-8-39.

CURCUMIN

Barry, et al. **Determining the Effects of Lipophilic Drugs on Membrane Structure by Solid-State NMR Spectroscopy: The Case of the Antioxidant Curcumin**. Journal of the American Chemical Society, 2009; 131 (12): 4490 DOI: 10.1021/ja809217u.

A. Masoumi, B. Goldenson, S. Ghirmai, H. Avagyan, J. Zaghi, K. Abel, et al. **1α,25-dihydroxyvitamin D3 Interacts with Curcuminoids to Stimulate Amyloid-β Clearance by Macrophages of Alzheimer's Disease Patients** Journal Of Alzheimer's Disease. Volume 17, Number 3, July 2009 Pages 703-717.

S. Jha, R. Patel. Some Observations on the Spectrum of Dementia. Neurol India 2004; 52:213-4.

ADAPT Research Group. **Cognitive Function Over Time in the Alzheimer's Disease Anti-inflammatory Prevention Trial (ADAPT): Results of a Randomized, Controlled Trial of Naproxen and Celecoxib** Arch Neurol, Jul 2008; 65: 896-905. DOI:10.1001/archneur.2008.65.7.nct70006.

DIABETES

P.L. Yau, D. C. Javier, C. M. Ryan, W. H. Tsui, B. A. Ardekani, S. Ten and A. Convit. **Preliminary Evidence for Brain Complications in Obese Adolescents with Type 2 Diabetes Mellitus.** Diabetologia, 2010; DOI: 10.1007/s00125-010-1857-y.

T. Matsuzaki, K. Sasaki, Y. Tanizaki, J. Hata, K. Fujimi, Y. Matsui, A. Sekita, S.O. Suzuki, S. Kanba, Y. Kiyohara, and T. Iwaki. **Insulin Resistance is Associated with the Pathology of Alzheimer Disease.** The Hisayama Study. Neurology, 2010; DOI: 10.1212/WNL.0b013e3181eee25f.

J.A. Sonnen, et al. **Different Patterns of Cerebral Injury in Dementia With or Without Diabetes.** Arch Neurol, 2009; 66 (3) DOI: 10.1001/archneurol.2008.579.

R.O. Roberts, et al. **Association of Duration and Severity of Diabetes Mellitus With Mild Cognitive Impairment.** Archives of Neurology, 2008; 65 (8): 1066 DOI: 10.1001/archneur.65.8.1066.

R.W. Gelling, et al. **Insulin Action in the Brain Contributes to Glucose Lowering During Insulin Treatment of Diabetes.** Cell Metabolism Vol. 3, Issue 1; January 2006, pages 67-73. DOI 10.1016/j.cmet.2005.11.013 www.cellmetabolism.org.

Weili Xu, et al. **Mid- and Late-Life Diabetes in Relation to the Risk of Dementia. Diabetes,** January 2009.

T. Cukierman-Yaffe, et al. **Relationship Between Baseline Glycemic Control and Cognitive Function in Individuals with Type 2 Diabetes and Other Cardiovascular Risk Factors: The Action to Control Cardiovascular Risk in Diabetes-Memory in Diabetes.** (ACCORD-MIND) trial. Diabetes Care, February 2009, 32:221-226; DOI:10.2337/dc08-1153.

A.M. Stranahan, T.V. Arumugam, R.G. Cutler, K. Lee, J.M. Egan and M.P. Mattson, **Diabetes Impairs Hippocampal Function Through Glucocorticoid-mediated Effects on New and Mature Neurons.** Nature Neuroscience, 11, 309 - 317 (2008) Published online: 17 February 2008, DOI:10.1038/nn2055.

EGGS

M.Q. Holmes-McNary, R. Loy, M-H. Mar, C.D. Albright and S.H. Zeisel. **Apoptosis is Induced by Choline Deficiency in Fetal Brain and PC12 Cells.** Developmental Brain Research, Vol. 101, Issue 1-2, July 1997, Pages 9-16. DOI: 10.1016/S0165-3806(97)00044-8.

Duke University Medical Centre (1998, April 9). **Extra Choline During Pregnancy Enhances Memory In Offspring.** ScienceDaily. Retrieved July 20 2010, from http://www.sciencedaily.com/releases/1998/04/980409080807.html.

EPIGENETICS

John Cloud. **Why Your DNA Isn't Your Destiny.** Time magazine, http://www.time.com/time/health/article/0,8599,1951968-1,00.html.

EXERCISE

Wu, et al. **Exercise Enhances the Proliferation of Neural Stem Cells and Neurite Growth and Survival of Neuronal Progenitor Cells in Dentate Gyrus of Middle-aged Mice.** Journal of Applied Physiology, 2008; 105 (5): 1585 DOI: 10.1152/japplphysiol.90775.2008.

L. Chaddock, K.I. Erickson, R.S. Prakash, J.S. Kim, M.W. Voss, M. Van Patter, et al. **A Neuroimaging Investigation of the Association Between Aerobic Fitness, Hippocampal Volume and Memory Performance in Preadolescent Children.** Brain Research, 2010; DOI: 10.1016/j.brainres.2010.08.049.

M.W. Voss, R.S. Prakash, K.I. Erickson, C. Basak, L. Chaddock, J.S. Kim, et al. **Plasticity of Brain Networks in a Randomized Intervention Trial of Exercise Training in Older Adults.** Frontiers in Aging Neuroscience, 2010; DOI: 10.3389/fnagi.2010.00032.

J.M. Burns, D.K. Johnson, A. Watts, R.H. Swerdlow, W.M. Brooks. **Reduced Lean Mass in Early Alzheimer Disease and Its Association With Brain Atrophy.** Arch Neurol, 2010; 67 (4): 428-433.

A. Bjornebekk, A.A. Mathe, S. Brene. **The Antidepressant Effect of Running is Associated with Increased Hippocampal Cell Proliferation** Int J Neuropsychopharmacol. 2005 Sep; 8(3):357-68.

N.T. Lautenschlager, et al. E**ffect of Physical Activity on Cognitive Function in Older Adults at Risk for Alzheimer Disease.** Journal of the American Medical Association, 2008; 300(9):1027-1037. DOI: 10.1001/jama.300.9.1027.

K.I. Erickson, R.S. Prakash, M.W. Voss, L. Chaddock, L. Hu, K.S. Morris, et al. Aerobic Fitness is Associated with Hippocampal Volume in Elderly Humans. Hippocampus, 2009; NA DOI: 10.1002/hipo.20547.

FISH

Rincón-Cervera, et al. **Fatty Acid Composition of Selected Roes from Some Marine Species.** European Journal of Lipid Science and Technology, 2009; 111 (9): 920 DOI: 10.1002/ejlt.200800256

A.D. Dangour, et al. **Effect of Long-chain Polyunsaturated Fatty Acid Supplementation on Cognitive Function in Older People: A Randomized, Double-blind, Controlled Trial.** Am. J. Clinical Nutrition, Apr 21, 2010 DOI: 10.3945/ajcn.2009.29121.

HOMOCYSTEINE

A.D. Smith, S.M. Smith , C.A. de Jager, P. Whitbread, C. Johnston, et al. 2010 **Homocysteine-Lowering by B Vitamins Slows the Rate of Accelerated Brain Atrophy in Mild Cognitive Impairment: A Randomized Controlled Trial.** PLoS ONE 5(9): e12244. DOI:10.1371/journal.pone.0012244.

HYPERTENSION

S. Oveisgharan; V. Hachinski. **Hypertension, Executive Dysfunction, and Progression to Dementia: The Canadian Study of Health and Aging.** Arch Neurol, 2010; 67 (2): 187-192.

C. Reitz, MD, PhD; M .Tang, PhD; J. Manly, PhD; R. Mayeux, MD, MSc; J.A. Luchsinger, MD, MPH. **Hypertension and the Risk of Mild Cognitive Impairment.** Arch Neurol. 2007; 64(12):1734-1740.

C. Lee, MD., W. Dai, PhD, J. Becker, PhD, L. Kuller, MD., H. Gach, PhD, et al. **Effects of Hypertension in Normal Aging, Mild Cognitive Impairment, and Alzheimer's Disease Evaluated with Arterial Spin Labeled MRI.** Paper presented at the annual meeting of the Radiological Society of North America (RSNA) 2007, November 29.

OBESITY AND CHOLESTEROL

A. C. Granholm, H.A. Bimonte-Nelson, A.B. Moore, M.E. Nelson, L.R. Freeman, K. Sambamurti. **Effects of a Saturated Fat and High Cholesterol Diet on Memory and Hippocampal Morphology in the Middle-Aged Rat.** Journal of Alzheimer's Disease, 14:2 (June 2008), pp. 133-145.

Stéphanie Debette, Alexa Beiser, Udo Hoffmann, Charles DeCarli, Christopher J. O'Donnell, Joseph M. Massaro, Rhoda Au, Jayandra J. Himali, Philip A. Wolf, Caroline S. Fox, Sudha Seshadri. **Visceral Fat is Associated with Lower Brain Volume in Healthy Middle-Aged Adults.** Annals of Neurology, August 2010; Volume 68, Issue 2, pages 136–144, DOI: 10.1002/ana.22062.

Gustafson, et al. **Adiposity Indicators and Dementia Over 32 Years in Sweden.** Neurology, 2009; 73 (19): 1559 DOI: 10.1212/WNL.0b013e3181c0d4b6.

JAMA and Archives Journals (2005, October 11). **Midlife Obesity May Be Associated With Risk Of Dementia And Alzheimer's Disease.** Arch Neurol. 2009; 66[3]:336-342.

RESVERATROL

Brown, et al. **The Biological Responses to Resveratrol and Other Polyphenols from Alcoholic Beverages.** Alcoholism Clinical and Experimental Research, 2009; DOI: 10.1111/j.1530-0277.2009.00989.

Sink, et al. **Moderate Alcohol Intake is Associated with Lower Dementia Incidence: Results from the Ginkgo Evaluation of Memory Study (GEMS).** Alzheimer's and Dementia, 2009; 5 (4): P105 DOI: 10.1016/j.jalz.2009.05.329.

SLEEP

A. Gohar, A. Adams, E. Gertner, L. Sackett-Lundeen, R. Heitz, R. Engle, E. Haus, J. Bijwadia. **Working Memory Capacity is Decreased in Sleep-deprived Internal Medicine Residents.** J Clin Sleep Med 2009;5(3):191-197.

G.R. Poe, C.M. Walsh, T.E. Bjorness. **Both Duration and Timing of Sleep are Important to Memory Consolidation.** Sleep. 2010 Oct 1;33(10):1277-8

M.A. Tucker, W. Fishbein. **Enhancement of Declarative Memory Performance Following a Daytime Nap Is Contingent on Strength of Initial Task Acquisition.** Sleep Volume 31, Issue 02.

E.A. Kensinger, J.D. Payne. **Sleep's Role in the Consolidation of Emotional Episodic Memories.** Current Directions in Psychological Science, October 12, 2010; Vol. 19 no. 5 290-295 doi: 10.1177/0963721410383978.

J.L. Gerrard, S.N. Burke, B.L. McNaughton, and C.A. Barnes. **Sequence Reactivation in the Hippocampus is Impaired in Aged Rats.** The Journal of Neuroscience, 30 July 2008, 28(31): 7883-7890; DOI: 10.1523/JNEUROSCI.1265-08.2008.

POSITIVE ATTITUDE

A.D. Ong. **Pathways Linking Positive Emotion and Health in Later Life.** Current Directions in Psychological Science, 2010; 19 (6): 358 DOI: 10.1177/0963721410388805.

Cohn, et al. **Happiness Unpacked: Positive Emotions Increase Life Satisfaction by Building Resilience.** Emotion, 2009; 9 (3): 361 DOI: 10.1037/a0015952.

M.A. Rapp, M. Schnaider-Beeri, H.T. Grossman, M. Sano, D.P. Perl, D.P. Purohit, et al. **Increased Hippocampal Plaques and Tangles in Patients With Alzheimer Disease With a Lifetime History of Major Depression.** Arch Gen Psychiatry. 2006;63:161-167.

MEDITATION

Katherine MacLean, Clifford Saron, B. Alan Wallace, et al. **Intensive Meditation Training Improves Perceptual Discrimination and Sustained Attention.** Psychological Science, June 2010 Vol. 21 no. 6 829-839.

Britta K. Hölzel, James Carmody, Mark Vangel, Christina Congleton, Sita M. Yerramsetti, Tim Gard, Sara W. Lazar. **Mindfulness Practice Leads to Increases in Regional Brain Gray Matter Density.** Psychiatry Research: Neuroimaging, 2011; 191 (1): 36 DOI: 10.1016/j.pscychresns.2010.08.006.

MEDITERRANEAN DIET

N. Scarmeas; Y. Stern; R. Mayeux; J.J. Manly; N. Schupf; J.A. Luchsinger. **Mediterranean Diet and Mild Cognitive Impairment.** Arch Neurol., 2009; 66 (2): 216-225.

J.M. Zhuo, D. Pratico. **Normalization of Hyperhomocysteinemia Improves Cognitive Deficits and Ameliorates Brain Amyloidosis of a Transgenic Mouse Model of Alzheimer's Disease.** The FASEB Journal, 2010; DOI: 10.1096/fj. 10-161828.

N. Scarmeas; J.A.Luchsinger; R.Mayeux; Y.Stern. **Mediterranean Diet and Alzheimer Mortality.** Neurology September 11, 2007, Vol. 69 no. 11 1084-1093 doi: 10.1212/01.wnl.0000277320.50685.7c.

VITAMIN D

L. Tripkovic et al **Comparison of vitamin D2 and vitamin D3 supplementation in raising serum 25-hydroxyvitamin D status: a systematic review and meta-analysis.** American Journal of Clinical Nutrition, 2012; 95 (6): 1357 DOI: 10.3945/ajcn.111.031070

W. B. Grant. **Does Vitamin D Reduce the Risk of Dementia?** Journal of Alzheimer's Disease, 17:1 (May 2009)

R. M. Lucas et al. **Sun exposure and vitamin D are independent risk factors for CNS demyelination.** Neurology, 2011; 76 (6): 540 DOI: 10.1212/WNL.0b013e31820af93d

E. E. Hohman et al. **Bioavailability and Efficacy of Vitamin D2 from UV-Irradiated Yeast in Growing, Vitamin D-Deficient Rats.** Journal of Agricultural and Food Chemistry, 2011; : 110218145952037 DOI: 10.1021/jf104679c

R. R. Simon, K. M. Phillips, R. L. Horst, I. C. Munro. **Vitamin D Mushrooms: Comparison of the Composition of Button Mushrooms (Agaricus bisporus) Treated Postharvest with UVB Light or Sunlight.** Journal of Agricultural and Food Chemistry, 2011; 59 (16): 8724 DOI: 10.1021/jf201255b

C. Karohl, et al. **Heritability and seasonal variability of vitamin D concentrations in male twins.** American Journal of Clinical Nutrition, 2010; DOI: 10.3945/ajcn.2010.30176

The International Osteoporosis Foundation http://www.osteofound.org

P. Knekt et al. **Serum Vitamin D and the Risk of Parkinson Disease.** Arch Neurol, 2010; 67 (7): 808-811

M. L. Evatt et al. **Prevalence of Vitamin D Insufficiency in Patients With Parkinson Disease and Alzheimer Disease.** Archives of Neurology, 2008; 65 (10): 1348 DOI: 10.1001/archneur.65.10.1348

M. L. Evatt. **Beyond Vitamin Status: Is There a Role for Vitamin D in Parkinson Disease?** Arch Neurol, 2010; 67 (7): 795-797

M. L. Evatt, et al. for the Parkinson Study Group DATATOP Investigators. **High Prevalence of Hypovitaminosis D Status in Patients With Early Parkinson Disease.** Arch Neurol, 2011; 68 (3): 314-319 DOI: 10.1001/archneurol.2011.30

I. Caesar et al. **Curcumin Promotes A-beta Fibrillation and Reduces Neurotoxicity in Transgenic Drosophila.** PLoS ONE, 2012; 7 (2): e31424 DOI: 10.1371/journal.pone.0031424

M. T. Mizwicki et al. **Genomic and Nongenomic Signaling Induced by 1α,25(OH)2-Vitamin D3 Promotes the Recovery of Amyloid-β Phagocytosis by Alzheimer's Disease Macrophages.** Journal Of Alzheimer's Disease. Volume 29, Number 1, March 2012 Pages 51-62

W. M. Panneton, V. B. Kumar, Qi Gan, W. J. Burke, J. E. Galvin. **The Neurotoxicity of DOPAL: Behavioral and Stereological Evidence for Its Role in Parkinson Disease Pathogenesis.** PLoS ONE, 2010; 5 (12): e15251 DOI: 10.1371/journal.pone.0015251

http://www.parkinsonswa.org.au/

D. K. Houston et al. **Low 25-Hydroxyvitamin D Predicts the Onset of Mobility Limitation and Disability in Community-Dwelling Older Adults: The Health ABC Study.** The Journals of Gerontology Series A: Biological Sciences and Medical Sciences, 2012; DOI: 10.1093/gerona/gls136

C. Annweiler et al. **Higher Vitamin D Dietary Intake Is Associated With Lower Risk of Alzheimer's Disease: A 7-Year Follow-up.** The Journals of Gerontology Series A: Biological Sciences and Medical Sciences, 2012; 67 (11): 1205 DOI: 10.1093/gerona/gls107

Y. Slinin et al. Association Between Serum 25(OH) **Vitamin D and the Risk of Cognitive Decline in Older Women**. The Journals of Gerontology Series A: Biological Sciences and Medical Sciences, 2012; 67 (10): 1092 DOI: 10.1093/gerona/gls075

The Peninsula College of Medicine and Dentistry (2009, January 24). **Low Levels Of Vitamin D Link To Problems In Older People.**

I. Shah et al. **Low 25OH Vitamin D2 Levels Found in Untreated Alzheimer's Patients, Compared to Acetylcholinesterase-Inhibitor Treated and Controls.** Current Alzheimer Research, 2012; 9 (9): 1069-1076

C. Annweiler., D.J. Llewellyn. and O. Beauchet. (2013) **Low serum vitamin d concentrations in Alzheimer's disease: a systematic review and meta-analysis.** J Alzheimers Dis. 1;33(3):659-74. doi: 10.3233/JAD-2012-121432.

Ganji et al (2010) **Serum Vitamin D concentrations are related to depression in young adult US population: the Third National Health and Nutrition Examination Survey.** International Archives of Medicine 3: 29 http://www.intarchmed.com/content/3/1/29

J. Maddock, D. J. Berry, M-C. Geoffroy, C. Power, E. Hyppönen (2013) **Vitamin D and common mental disorders in mid-life: Cross-sectional and prospective findings.** Clinical Nutrition (10.1016/j.clnu.2013.01.006)

T Bowerman, S. Thomas. J. Mullan, M. Reeves. **Vitamin D deficiency in the elderly: How can we improve rates of screening and supplementation in General Practice?** Australian Medical Student Journal v3 i1 pp23-26